Instructor's Guide for

W9-ADI-997

Clinical Applications of Nursing Diagnosis:

Adult, Child, Women's, Psychiatric,
Gerontic, and Home Health Considerations

Third Edition

Helen C. Cox, RN, C, EdD, FAAN
Mittie D. Hinz, RNC, MSN
Mary Ann Lubno, RN, PhD, CNAA
Susan A. Newfield, RN, MSN, CS
Nancy A. Ridenour, RN, PhD, CFNC, FAAN
Mary McCarthy Slater, RN, C, MSN
Kathryn L. Sridaromont, RNC, MSN

 F. A. Davis Company • Publishers

F. A. Davis Company
1915 Arch Street
Philadelphia, PA 19103

Last digit indicates print number: 10 9 8 7 6 5 4 3 2 1

Printed in the United States of America

ISBN
0 - 8036 - 0178 - 6

CONTENTS

Part I   Why This Book?, 1

Part II   Book Organization, 4

Part III   How To Use This Book, 9

Part IV   Admission Assessment, 13

Part V   Developing Expected Outcomes, 67

Case Study 1   Chris Appleton, 101

Case Study 2   Ann Bastrow, 112

Case Study 3   Fred Carson, 122

Case Study 4   Betty Dawmer, 131

Case Study 5   Jessica Keymeyer, 139

Case Study 6   Emma Watson, 148

Case Study 7   Joseph Wilson, 159

Case Study 8   David Patterson, 171

Case Study 9   Roger Dalton, 180

Case Study 10   Charles Dean, 188

Part VI   Transparency Masters, 195

PART I-WHY THIS BOOK

The notion and content for this book were born, as you might have experienced also, through frustration with the currently available books regarding Nursing Diagnosis. The faculty at our various authors' schools are highly supportive of the work of the North American Nursing Diagnosis Association (NANDA). This support is based on the belief that the use of NANDA Nursing Diagnosis helps to define the essence of nursing and gives direction to care that is uniquely Nursing Care. As instructors we also found the need to give students consistency and direction when choosing to use a Nursing Diagnosis. What better to work with than the well defined standards that NANDA provides.

Due to the support for and belief in the work of NANDA, we wished to start our basic students out working with the concept of Nursing Diagnosis and continue this study throughout their schooling. Our curriculum arrangement required a very basic book that could be used as a teaching tool and as a reference book for our students. Thus our first reason for writing this book was to provide a level of presentation that could be used by any student (ADN, DIPL or BSN) or practicing nurse who was totally unfamiliar with Nursing Diagnosis.

A second concern we had related to the number of books students needed to purchase throughout the length of a program. As they progressed through different clinical areas, they found the need for various new clinical references. In some cases the availability of such books were neither affordable nor suitable to their purposes. The majority of the currently published books focus on adult health with limited information about the other areas of pediatric, mental-psychiatric health, obstetrical-gynecological, gerontic or home health nursing.

Additionally, in the currently available literature, there is limited information regarding physiological, psychological, sociological, and developmental content. All of which could significantly impact the delivery of care based on nursing diagnosis. These factors can greatly influence the choice and implementation of any Nursing Diagnosis especially when considering the adaptation of care required for different stages of the developmental cycle.

We found our students were bringing a variety of references to the clinical sites to assist in planning care for their individual patient. Some of these included care planning, A & P, and age span development books. While we make clinical assignments the day before the scheduled clinical practice and expect the students to be prepared, the students brought the books for what they termed "in cases". In case the patient had been discharged before the student arrived for clinical practice. In case the patient's condition had changed and new diagnoses were needed. In case the student's original diagnosis was wrong and needed to be revised and as one student succinctly stated, "Just generally in case". Therefore we designed this book to help the students meet this particular need for readily available and comprehensive information in one book.

A third concern we had was our desire to focus on concepts rather than specifics. We have never met a faculty member teaching who believes there is sufficient time to teach everything a student needs to learn to begin practice. We have chosen to deal with this problem by focusing on concepts. Several previously published books use nursing diagnosis to contribute to nursing care plans. However, these books focus outcome and nursing interventions on the etiologies, causative or other factors that result in the Nursing

2

Diagnosis. We have chosen to focus Nursing Intervention on the Nursing Diagnosis itself. To focus on the Nursing Diagnosis promotes the use of concepts in nursing rather than worrying about a multitude of specifics.

For example, there are common interventions for pain regardless of whether the etiological factor is surgery, a fracture, labor, or neurological dysfunction. Using the conceptual approach also does away with the arguments of "Can a medical diagnosis be used as a related factor?" and "Can a Nursing Diagnosis be used as a related factor for another Nursing Diagnosis?"

Finally, we are led to what could easily be argued as the single most important factor in our decision to write this book. Reviewing all the books on the market which focus on Nursing Diagnosis and/or Care Planning, you will see that only the first four steps, assessment, diagnosis, planning and intervention, of the Nursing Process are covered. Evaluation, this final and truly important step is nowhere to be found. Yet we all teach our students to think and perform nursing activities via this process.

As authors of this text, we have provided our readers a basic introduction to this extremely important phase of the Nursing Process. By using Algorithms (or Flowcharts), the reader can follow a series of yes and no queries pertaining to patient's progress toward achieving the expected outcome.

These are the concerns that led us to writing this book. We are pleased with our student's response to the book and the very positive feedback they have given about its helpfulness and utility. Our wish is you will also find the book of value to you and your students.

PART II - BOOK ORGANIZATION

We chose Marjory Gordon's Functional Health Patterns as the organizational framework for the book. Gordon identified the functional health patterns circa 1974 to assist in the teaching of assessment and diagnosis at the Boston College School of Nursing. The title of each Functional Health Pattern is, in essence, self-explanatory. This makes the patterns extremely easy to use.

Additionally, Functional Health Patterns allow grouping of the nursing diagnoses into mutually inclusive sets which, in our opinion, promotes a conceptual approach to assessment and selection of a Nursing Diagnosis. The NANDA typology, Human Response Patterns, is still in the initial stages of development and does not provide mutually inclusive groupings as clearly as Gordon's patterns. Because the patterns were developed to assist in teaching and because the diagnoses can be placed in mutually inclusive categories, we believe the use of Gordon's Functional Health Patterns facilitates teaching and learning about Nursing Diagnosis.

Provided for each Functional Health Pattern is a pattern introduction which includes a pattern description, a pattern assessment, conceptual information, and developmental considerations. The pattern description provides a definition of the pattern and gives a short succinct discussion of the overall content of the pattern.

The pattern assessment gives factors that should be used as a guide in determining if the particular pattern is pertinent for this patient. Using the pattern assessment first, saves the student time in assessing for individual Nursing Diagnoses. (If the patient demonstrated signs and symptoms related to the pattern, then the student knows to go to individual diagnosis assessment. If the patient demonstrates no signs or symptoms related to the pattern then the student can progress to another pattern assessment without being concerned about missing a Nursing Diagnosis.)

The conceptual information section has been briefly discussed under the reasons for writing this book. The conceptual information includes physiological, psychological, and sociological content related to the entire Functional Health Pattern and provides a "quick reference" review of the content for the student.

Developmental considerations focus on the evolutionary milestones for each of the following age groups: infant, toddler and pre-schooler, school-aged, adolescent, young adult, adult and older adult. The developmental considerations give assistance to the student by pointing out factors that might need adjustment due to the developmental level of the client.

Following all the information regarding the Pattern Introduction is a section title Applicable Nursing Diagnoses. This section includes the individual Nursing Diagnoses categorized in that pattern. Each diagnosis within the pattern is listed in alphabetic order. Modifiers for each diagnosis, such as altered, risk, impaired, ineffective and actual, are separated from the diagnosis by a comma and the diagnosis itself is placed in alphabetical order. (e.g., Cardiac Output, Altered; Physical Mobility, Impaired; and Infection, Risk for.)

For each individual diagnosis the following information is included: definition, defining characteristics, related factors, related clinical concerns, a validity check titled "Have you selected the correct diagnosis?", expected outcomes, target date, nursing actions/interventions with rationales (adult health, child health, women's health, mental health, gerontic health and home health), and evaluation.

To promote the development of NANDA's work and to promote consistency in communication, we use NANDA's definitions, defining characteristics, and related factors. F.A. Davis provided a grant to NANDA to permit our use of this material. Other books use their own versions of these items! We believe this leads to confusion for the students and does not assist NANDA in refining their work.

Diagnosis validation (Have you selected the correct diagnosis?) is included as a resource in aiding the student in selecting an appropriate Nursing Diagnosis. The information included in this section shows the student how to discern such closely related diagnoses as Self-Care Deficit and Altered Health Maintenance, Ineffective Thermoregulation and Hyperthermia or Hypothermia, and Anxiety and Fear. Use of the validation section promotes the student's confidence in working with Nursing Diagnosis as well as enhances a student's actual understanding of that diagnosis.

At least two expected outcomes are given for each and every diagnosis. The expected outcomes are worded in behavioral, measurable, patient-oriented terms. The proper wording of expected outcomes serves as the base for the evaluation stage. Connected to the expected outcome is a target date. The target date helps in pacing the plan of care, assists both the patient and the nurse to see accomplishments and, most importantly, alerts the student when to evaluate the plan of care. The target date does not mean the expected outcome must be totally met, but instead signals when to evaluate progress toward meeting the expected outcome. The target date also helps insure that the plan of care is kept current. Included in this manual, as Part IV, is a short programmed unit on "Developing Expected Outcomes". This unit will teach the student, in a rapid manner, how to correctly write behaviorally stated expected outcomes that focus on patient action.

Nursing actions/interventions with appropriate rationales are given for Adult Health (Med-Surg), Child Health (Peds), Women's Health (OB/GYN, neonate), Mental Health (Psych), Gerontic Health and Home Health. The adult health nursing actions serve as the generic actions, in most diagnoses, with the other sections denoting the possible adaptations necessary for the clinical area or a patient's age. Nursing actions are stated in terms of nurse behavior and, as appropriate, are stated specific with time periods, frequency, and so forth. It is our philosophy that nursing actions need to be as directive as physician's orders to increase better communication and consistency for the patient's care. Rationales were included to assist the student in understanding the basic reason(s) that led to the inclusion of the particular nursing action in the plan of care. While we tried to include as many scientific rationales as possible some of the rationales reflect basic common sense rationales that are the backbone of nursing care.

Evaluation is presented in the form of algorithms or Flowcharts. As previously indicated, evaluation is based on the stated expected outcome. In the evaluation flow, the student starts by asking a simple yes/no question related to the expected outcome. Based on whether the answer is yes or no, pathways are given to assist the student in arriving at a decision in regards to the patient's progress and a decision about revising the plan of care. The plan of care decisions include revise, continue, and resolved. REVISE can mean changing a previous diagnosis or adding a new diagnosis based on evaluation data collection. CONTINUE indicates keeping the same diagnosis, adding to the nursing actions as necessary and changing the target date. RESOLVED means the Nursing Diagnosis no longer exists, the patient's problem has been taken care of. The algorithms also give the student an indication of what data should be collected to validate the evaluation decision.

In some instances, additional information is included. The additional information includes material that either needs to be highlighted or does not logically fall within the defined outline areas.

References are given at the end of the book and are arranged according to each chapter. To provide the student the broadest possible range of assistive information, both textbooks and journal articles are included.

PART III - HOW TO USE THIS BOOK

The information in this section is based on our experiences teaching Nursing Diagnosis to our students and workshop participants. While these suggestions work well within our particular curriculum, some adjustments may be necessary for your particular program.

We set out by focusing the student's attention to the Preface and Chapter 1–the Overview. This familiarizes the student with the general concepts and premises underlying the entire book. The preface and Chapter 1 also explains how to translate the five-part Nursing process into an active care plan and gives them a thorough introduction to each phase of the nursing plan of care. By using the example provided in the book, we sketch a care plan form on the chalkboard and enter the data as we progress through the chapter. Demonstration is also given on the chalkboard regarding the use of the nursing actions as a guide for documentation (Also given as an example in Chapter 1). By utilizing the section Valuing Care Planning we emphasize the importance of plans of care and start the students' thinking about how they could promote the use of care planning in the clinical agencies. We demonstrate to the student how the recent changes in JCAHO standards regarding care plans can be implemented using a variety of documentation formats such as problem oriented charting, FOCUS charting, PIE charting, and the like. It is important to remind the students while JCAHO did say the agency no longer had to have a separate form for the plan of care, the care plan must still be reflected in the health care record. The care plan can be incorporated into documentation by such charting methods mentioned above.

After our discussion of the Preface and Chapter 1, we then proceed to the information on the Functional Health Patterns. We begin by citing Figure 1-3 (page 13) which gives the pattern labels and a brief description. From this figure we progress to the first page of each chapter from Chapters 2 to 11. We emphasize the pattern description and pattern assessment at this time.

To teach the remainder of the content, we utilize case studies. Examples of the case studies are given in Part VI of this manual. In teaching the student to transfer from the case study to patients, we begin by reviewing the admission assessment (Part IV of this manual, along with an example) and pattern description then go to the pattern assessment. In the pattern assessment data are validated by yes/no type questions. The yes/no questions incorporate both objective and subjective data and point the student towards appropriate individual nursing diagnoses.

For the individual Nursing Diagnosis, the students review both the defining characteristics and the related factors (etiologies). At least 70% of the defining characteristics should be present and the related factors must be relevant for the diagnosis to be accepted for the patient.

In working with the case studies, each student is given a copy of all the studies to be used that day. The students are then divided into groups with each group being assigned responsibility for a different case. The groups work on the individual diagnoses first. Each group reports to the entire class on the diagnoses selected for their case study. (Students should be encouraged to keep notes on the diagnoses selected for the other case studies.) Faculty also interject questioning at this time to call attention to the validation content (Have you selected the correct diagnosis?) and offer further clarification and explanation as needed. Since validation content in this manner is unique to this book, you will be able to cite exactly where the rationale for this judgment is found within the chapter the students are utilizing.

Next, the groups are assigned work on the expected outcome(s) and target date for each diagnosis they have identified. (We make sure the students have completed the programmed unit and then have them write their own expected outcomes rather than using the ones in the text.) After the groups have shared their expected outcomes we go to the appropriate pages in the book to compare their stated expected outcomes to the expected outcome in the text. During comparison time, we stress behavioral statements, how to make them measurable, and emphasize realistic target dates.

The students are referred to the appropriate pages in the book to do group work on nursing actions. The faculty member's role at this time is to review the conceptual and developmental information to assist the student in understanding how this information can assist in adapting the plan of care to meet individual client needs. Following this review, we ask the students about rationales for the nursing actions and require them to answer without referring to the text. We then go back and compare their rationales to those give in the text.

A follow-up is provided for each case study so the student can have experience with evaluation. The students are urged to follow the algorithm flow in the book to learn at least one form of decision making. Again, each group shares with the class so all can benefit from following each others evaluation decisions as well as the actions following the decisions. This book is the only one available that speaks directly to teaching the most neglected phase of the Nursing Process—evaluation.

While we have found this method of using the text valuable to us, your curriculum arrangement may required a different method. The content can be taught going through the book chapter by chapter or by focusing on Chapter One related to nursing process and then skipping to chapters appropriate to your curriculum. It is also possible to teach Chapter One and then use a grouping of chapters, such as saving the chapters related to Coping-Stress Tolerance, Self-Perception-Self- Concept, and Role-Relationship for a course related to psychiatric/mental health nursing. Individual nursing diagnoses can also be assigned to certain courses, for example, you might wish to use all the Breastfeeding diagnoses only in maternal-child health, with the remaining diagnoses in that chapter being used in an adult health course. Remember Gordon's Functional Health Patterns are designed to be used as an organizing framework for assessment. The Functional Health Patterns are not designed to be a theory of nursing or a curriculum framework. The advantage to the Functional Health Patterns is, that being mutually inclusive, they are adaptable to use in a variety of curricula frameworks.

The authors very much enjoyed putting together this book. We have found it extremely valuable for our students and have received much positive feedback from the other schools of nursing who have employed it as a teaching text. It is our sincere desire that you and your students find it beneficial as well. Please feel free to share your input with us and F. A. Davis Company so we can continue to improve the book.

PART IV

ADMISSION ASSESSMENT

DEMOGRAPHIC DATA

Date:_____Time:_____

Name:_____

D.O.B.:_____ Age:_____

Sex:_____

Primary Significant Other:_____Telephone #_____

Name of Primary Information Source:_____

Admitting Medical Diagnosis_____

VITAL SIGNS

Temperature_____ F__C__ Oral__ Rectal__ Axillary__ Tympanic__

Pulse Rate: Radial_____ Apical_____; Regular__ Irregular__

Respiratory Rate_____ Abdominal__ Diaphragmatic__

Blood Pressure: Left Arm_____; Right Arm_____; Sitting__ Standing__ Lying

Down__

Weight_____ pounds, _____kilogram; Height: ___feet___inches, _____meters.

Do you have any allergies? No__ Yes__ What?_____

(Check reactions to medications, foods, cosmetics, insect bites, etc.)

Review admission CBC, Urinalyses, and Chest X-ray. Note any abnormalities here:

_____

HEALTH PERCEPTION/HEALTH MANAGEMENT PATTERN

Subjective

1. How would you describe your usual health status? Good__ Fair__ Poor__

2. Are you satisfied with your usual health status? Yes__ No__Source of

    Dissatisfaction_____

3. Tobacco Use? No__ Yes__ Number of packs per day_____

4. Alcohol Use? No__ Yes__ How much and what kind?_____

5. Street Drug Use? No__ Yes__ What_____

6. Any history of chronic diseases? No__ Yes__ What_____

    _____

7. Immunization History: Tetanus_____; Pneumonia_____;

    Influenza_____;MMR_____; Polio_____; Hepatitis B_____; Hib_____

8. Have you sought any health care assistance in the past year? No__ Yes__

    If yes, why?_____

9. Are you currently working? Yes__ No__ How would you rate your working

    conditions (e.g., safety, noise, space, heating, cooling, water, ventilation)?

    Excellent__ Good__ Fair__ Poor__ Describe any problems areas_____

    _____

10. How would you rate living conditions at home? Excellent__ Good__ Fair__

    Poor__ Describe any problem areas_____

11. Do you have any difficulty securing any of the following services?

    Grocery Store? Yes__ No__; Pharmacy? Yes__ No__;

    Health Care Facility? Yes__ No__; Transportation? Yes__ No__;

    Telephone (for police, fire, ambulance, etc.)? Yes__ No__;

If any difficulties, note referral here_____

12. Medications (Over-the-Counter and Prescriptive)

NAME   DOSAGE AMT. TIMES/DAY REASON TAKING AS

ORDERED

_____Yes__No__

_____Yes__No__

_____Yes__No__

_____Yes__No__

_____Yes__No__

_____Yes__No__

_____Yes__No__

_____Yes__No__

13. Have you followed the routine prescribed for you? Yes__ No__

Why not?_____

14. Did you think this prescribed routine was the best for you? Yes__ No__

What would be better?_____

15. Have you had any accidents/injuries/falls in the past year? No__ Yes__

Describe_____

16. Have you had any problems with cuts healing? No__ Yes__

Describe_____

17. Do you exercise on a regular basis? No__ Yes__ Type and Frequency____

_____

18. Have you experienced any ringing in the ears? Right - Yes__ No__

Left - Yes__ No__

19. Have you experienced any vertigo? Yes__ No__ How often and when____

_____

20. Do you regularly use seat belts? Yes___ No___

21. For infants and children, are car seats used regularly? Yes___ No___

22. Do you have any suggestions or assistance requests for improving your

    health ? No__ Yes__

23. Do you do (breast/testicular) self examination? No__ Yes__

    How often?_____

24. Were you or your family able to meet all your therapeutic needs? Yes__ No__

25. Are you scheduled for surgery? Yes__ No__

26. Have you recently had surgery? No__ Yes__ Date_____

Objective

1. Mental Status (Indicate assessment with an X)

    a. Oriented__ Disoriented__ Length of time_____

       Time: Yes__ No__ Length of time_____

       Place: Yes__ No__ Length of time_____

       Person: Yes__ No__ Length of time_____

    b. Sensorium

       Alert__; Drowsy__; Lethargic__; Stuporous__; Comatose__;

       Cooperative__; Combative__; Delusions__; Fluctuating levels of

       consciousness? Yes__ No__

       Appropriate response to stimuli? Yes__ No__

    c. Memory

       Recent? Yes__ No__; Remote? Yes__ No__; Past 4 hours? Yes__ No__

d. Is there a disruption of the flow of energy surrounding the person? Yes__

No__Change in color? Yes__ No__; Change in temperature? Yes__

No__;

Field? Yes__ No__; Movement? Yes__ No__; Sound? Yes__ No__

e. Responds to simple directions? Yes__ No__

2. Vision

a. Visual Acuity: Both eyes 20/___ Right 20/___ Left 20/___ Not

assessed__

b. Pupil Size: Right - Normal__ Abnormal; Left - Normal__ Abnormal__

Description of abnormalities_____

c. Pupil Reaction: Right - Normal__ Abnormal__; Left - Normal_

Abnormal__Description of Abnormalities_____

d. Wears Glasses? Yes__ No__; Contact Lenses? Yes__ No__

3. Hearing: Not assessed__

a. Right - WNL__ Impaired__ Deaf__; Left - WNL__ Impaired__ Deaf__

b. Hearing Aid? Yes__ No__

4. Taste

a. Sweet: Normal__ Abnormal__

Describe_____

b. Sour: Normal__ Abnormal__

Describe_____

c. Tongue Movement: Normal__ Abnormal__

Describe_____

d. Tongue Appearance: Normal__ Abnormal__

17

Describe_____

5. Touch

    a.   Blunt: Normal__ Abnormal__

        Describe_____

    b.   Sharp: Normal__ Abnormal__

        Describe_____

    c.   Light Touch Sensation: Normal__ Abnormal__

        Describe_____

    d.   Proprioception: Normal__ Abnormal__

        Describe_____

    e.   Heat: Normal__ Abnormal__

        Describe_____

    f.   Cold: Normal__ Abnormal__

        Describe_____

    g.   Any Numbness? No__ Yes__

        Describe_____

    h.   Any Tingling? No__ Yes__

        Describe_____

6. Smell

    a.   Rt Nostril: Normal__ Abnormal__

        Describe_____

    b.   Lt Nostril: Normal__ Abnormal__

        Describe_____

7. Assess Cranial Nerves: Normal__ Abnormal___

Describe deviations_____

8. Cerebellar Exam (Romberg, Balance, Gait, Coordination, etc.): Normal__

   Abnormal__Describe_____

   Assess Reflexes: Normal__ Abnormal__ Describe_____

   _____

10. Throat: Enlarged tonsils? No__ Yes__ Location _____

    Tenderness? No__ Yes__ Exudate on tonsils? No__ Yes__ Color_____

    Uvula midline? No__ Yes__

11. Neck: Any enlarged lymph nodes? No__ Yes__Location and size_____

    _____

12. General Appearance

    a   Hair_____

    b.   Skin_____

    c.   Nails_____

    d.   Body Odor_____

NUTRITIONAL/METABOLIC PATTERN

Subjective

1. Any weight gain in last 6 months? No__ Yes__ Amount_____

2. Any weight loss in last 6 months? No__ Yes__ Amount_____

3. Would you describe your appetite as: Good__ Fair__ Poor__

4. Do you have any food intolerances? No__ Yes__ Describe_____

    _____

5. Do you have any dietary restrictions? (Check for those that are a part of a prescribed regimen as well as those patient restricts voluntarily; e.g., to prevent flatus.) No__ Yes__ What_____

6. Describe an average day's food intake for you (meals and snacks)

_____

_____

_____

_____

_____

7. Describe an average day's fluid intake for you_____

_____

8. Describe food likes and dislikes_____

_____

9. Would you like to: Gain weight__ Lose weight__ Neither__

10. Any problems with:

  a. Nausea? No__ Yes__ Describe_____

  b. Vomiting? No__ Yes__ Describe_____

  c. Swallowing? No__ Yes__ Describe_____

  d. Chewing? No__ Yes__ Describe_____

  e. Indigestion? No__ Yes__ Describe_____

11. Would you describe your usual lifestyle as: Active__ Sedate__

For breastfeeding mothers only:

12. Do you have any concerns about breastfeeding? No__ Yes__

  Describe_____

13.   Are you having any problems with breastfeeding? No__ Yes__

Describe_____

Objective

1.   Skin Examination

    a.   Warm__; Cool__; Moist__; Dry__

    b.   Lesions? No__ Yes__ Describe_____

    c.   Rash? No__ Yes__ Describe_____

    d.   Turgor: Firm__; Supple__; Dehydrated__; Fragile__

        e.   Color: Pale__; Pink__; Dusky__; Cyanotic__; Jaundiced__;

        Mottled__; Other_____

2.   Mucous Membranes

    a.   Mouth

        (1)   Moist__ Dry__

        (2)   Lesions? No__ Yes__ Describe_____

        (3)   Color: Pale__ Pink__

        (4)   Teeth: Normal__ Abnormal__ Describe_____

        (5)   Dentures? No__ Yes__ Upper__ Lower__ Partial__

        (6)   Gums: Normal__ Abnormal__ Describe_____

        (7)   Tongue: Normal__ Abnormal__ Describe_____

    b.   Eyes

        (1)   Moist__ Dry__

        (2)   Color of conjunctiva: Pale__ Pink__ Jaundiced__

        (3)   Lesions? No__ Yes__ Describe_____

5.   Edema

a.   General? No__ Yes__ Describe_____

_____

Abdominal Girth _____inches; Not measured__

b.   Periorbital? No__ Yes__ Describe_____

c.   Dependent? No__ Yes__ Describe_____

Ankle Girth: Right _____inches; Left _____inches; Not measured__

6.   Thyroid: Normal__ Abnormal__ Describe_____

7.   Jugular Vein Distention? No__ Yes__

8.   Gag Reflex: Present__ Absent__

9.   Can patient move self easily (turning, walking)? Yes__ No__

Describe limitations_____

10.   Upon admission was patient dressed appropriately for the weather? Yes__

No__ Describe_____

For Breastfeeding Mothers Only

11.   Breast Exam: Normal__ Abnormal__ Describe_____

_____

12.   Weigh infant. Is infant's weight within normal limits? Yes__ No__

ELIMINATION PATTERN

Subjective

1.   What is your usual frequency of bowel movements? _____

a.   Have to strain to have BM? No__ Yes__

b.   Same time each day? No__ Yes__

2.   Has the number of bowel movements changed in the past week? No__ Yes__

Increased__ Decreased__

3. Character of stool:

    a.   Consistency: Hard__ Soft__ Liquid__

    b.   Color: Brown__ Black__ Yellow__ Clay colored__

    c.   Bleeding with bowel movements? No__ Yes__

4. History of constipation? No__ Yes__ How often_____

    Use bowel movement aids (laxatives, suppositories, diet)? No__ Yes__

    Describe_____

5. History of diarrhea? No__ Yes__ When_____

6. History of Incontinence? No__ Yes__

    Related to increased abdominal pressure (coughing, laughing, sneezing)? No__

        Yes__

7. History of recent travel? No__ Yes__ Where_____

8. Usual voiding pattern:

    a.   Frequency (times/day)_____ Decreased__ Increased__

    b.   Change in Awareness of Need to Void? No__ Yes__

        Increased__ Decreased__

    c.   Change in Urge to Void? No__ Yes__ Increased__ Decreased__

    b.   Any Change in Amount? No__ Yes__ Decreased__ Increased__

    c.   Color: Yellow__ Smokey__ Dark__

    d.   Incontinence? No__ Yes__When_____

        Difficulty holding voiding when urge to void develops? No__Yes__

        Have time to get to bathroom? Yes__ No__

        How often does problem reaching bathroom occur_____

    e.   Retention? No__ Yes__ Describe_____

f.   Pain/burning? No___ Yes___ Describe_____

g.   Sensation of bladder spasms? No___ Yes___ When_____

Objective

1.   Auscultate abdomen.

      a.   Bowel Sounds: Normal___ Increased___ Decreased___ Absent___

2.   Palpate abdomen.

      a.   Tender? No___ Yes___ Where?_____

      b.   Soft? Yes___ No___; Firm? Yes___ No___

      c.   Masses? No___ Yes___ Describe_____

      d.   Distention (include distended bladder)? No___ Yes___ Describe____

_____

      e.   Overflow urine when bladder palpated? Yes___ No___

3.   Rectal Exam

      a.   Sphincter tone: Describe_____

      b.   Hemorrhoids? No___ Yes___ Describe_____

      c.   Stool in rectum? No___ Yes___ Describe_____

      d.   Impaction? No___ Yes___ Describe_____

      e.   Occult Blood? No___ Yes___

4.   Ostomy Present? No___ Yes___ Location_____

ACTIVITY-EXERCISE PATTERN

Subjective

1.   Using the Functional Level Classification below have patient rate each area of self care. (Code adapted by NANDA from E. Jones, et al. Patient Classification for

Long-Term care: Users' Manual, HEW, Publication No. HRA-74-3107. November, 1974).

0 = Completely independent

1 = Requires use of equipment or device.

2 = Requires help from another person, for assistance, supervision, or teaching.

3 = Requires help from another person and equipment device.

4 = Dependent, does not participate in activity.

Feeding _____; Bathing/Hygiene _____; Dressing/Grooming_____;

Toileting_____; Ambulation_____; Care of home_____; Shopping____;

Meal preparation_____; Laundry_____; Transportation_____.

2.   Oxygen use at home? No__ Yes__ Describe_____

3.   How many pillows do you use to sleep on: Number_____

4.   Do you frequently experience fatigue? No__ Yes__ Describe_____

_____

5.   How many stairs can you climb without experiencing any difficulty?

       Number (can be individual number or number of flights) _____

6.   How far can you walk without experiencing any difficulty? _____

7.   Has assistance at home for care of self and maintenance of home? No__ Yes__

       Who_____

       If No, would like to have or believes needs to have assistance? No__Yes__

       With What Activities_____

8.   Occupation (if retired, former occupation)_____

9.   Describe your usual leisure time activities/hobbies_____

10. Any complaints of weakness or lack of energy? No__ Yes__

Describe_____

11. Any difficulties in maintaining activities of daily living? No__ Yes__

Describe_____

12. Any problems with concentration? No__ Yes__ Describe_____

Objective

1. Cardiovascular

 a. Cyanosis? No__ Yes__ Where_____

 b. Pulses: Easily palpable?

 Carotid--Yes__ No__; Jugular--Yes__ No__; Temporal--Yes__ No__;

 Radial--Yes__ No__; Femoral--Yes__ No__; Popliteal--Yes__ No__;

 Post Tibial--Yes__ No__; Dorsalis pedis--Yes__ No__.

 c. Extremities:

 (1) Temperature: Cold__ Cool__ Warm__ Hot__

 (2) Capillary Refill: Normal__ Delayed__

 (3) Color: Pink__ Pale__ Cyanotic__ Other__

 Describe_____

 (4) Homan's Sign? No__ Yes__

 (5) Nails: Normal__ Abnormal__ Describe_____

 (6) Hair Distribution: Normal__ Abnormal__ Describe_____

 _____

 (7) Claudication? No__ Yes__ Describe_____

d. Heart: PMI Location_____

    (1) Abnormal rhythm? No__ Yes__ Describe_____

    _____

    (2) Abnormal sounds? No__ Yes__ Describe_____

    _____

2. Respiratory

a. Rate_____; Depth - Shallow__ Deep__ Abdominal__

    Diaphragmatic__

b. Have patient cough. Any sputum? No__ Yes__ Describe_____

    _____

c. Fremitus? No__ Yes__

d. Any chest excursion? No__ Yes__ Equal__ Unequal__

e. Ausculatate Chest:

    Any abnormal sounds (Rales, Rhonchi)? No__ Yes__

    Describe_____

f. Have pt. walk in place for 3 minutes (if permissible):

    (1) Any shortness of breath after activity? No__ Yes__

    (2) Any dyspnea? No__ Yes__

    (3) B.P. after activity_____/_____ in (Rt; Left) arm.

    (4) Respiratory rate after activity_____

    (5) Pulse rate after activity_____

3. Musculo-Skeletal

a. Range of motion: Normal__ Limited__ Describe_____

b. Gait: Normal__ Abnormal__ Describe_____

c. Balance: Normal__ Abnormal__ Describe_____

d. Muscle Mass/Strength: Normal__ Increased__ Decreased__

Describe_____

e. Hand Grasp: Right - Normal__ Decreased__

Left - Normal__ Decreased__

f. Toe Wiggle: Right - Normal__ Decreased__

Left - Normal__ Decreased__

g. Posture: Normal__ Kyphosis__ Lordosis__

h. Deformities? No__ Yes__ Describe_____

i. Missing limbs? No__ Yes__ Where_____

j. Uses mobility assistive devices (walker, crutches, etc.)? No__ Yes__

Describe_____

k. Tremors? No__ Yes__ Describe_____

l. Traction or Casts present? No__ Yes__ Describe_____

4. Spinal Cord Injury? No__ Yes__ Level_____

5. Paralysis present? No__ Yes__ Where_____

6. Conduct developmental assessment. Normal__ Abnormal__ Describe_____

_____

7. Responds appropriately to stimuli? Yes__ No__ Describe_____

_____

8. Are there any abnormal movements? No__ Yes__ Describe_____

_____

SLEEP-REST PATTERN

Subjective

1. Usual sleep habits: Hours/night_____; Naps? No__ Yes__ AM__ PM__

   Feel rested? Yes__ No__ Describe_____

2. Any problems:

   a. Difficulty going to sleep? No__ Yes__

   b. Awakening during night? No__ Yes__

   c. Early awakening? No__ Yes__

   d. Insomnia? No__ Yes__ Describe_____

3. Methods used to promote sleep: Medication? No__ Yes__ Name_____

   Warm fluids? No__ Yes__ What_____

   Relaxation techniques? No__ Yes__

Objective

None

COGNITIVE-PERCEPTUAL PATTERN

Subjective

1. Pain.

   a. Location (have pt. point to)_____

   b. Intensity (have pt. rank on scale of 0-10)_____

   c. Radiation? No__ Yes__ To where_____

   d. Timing (how often; related to any specific events)_____

      _____

   e. Duration_____

   f. What do to relieve at home_____

   g. When did pain begin_____

2. Decision Making

a. Find decision making: Easy__ Moderately easy__ Moderately difficult__ Difficult__

b. Inclined to make decisions: Rapidly__ Slowly__ Delay__

c. Difficulty choosing between options? Yes__ No__ Describe_____

_____

3. Knowledge level

a. Can define what current problem is? Yes__ No__

b. Can restate current therapeutic regimen? Yes__ No__

Objective

1. Review sensory and mental status completed in Health Perception-Health Management Pattern.

2. Any overt signs of pain? No__ Yes__ Describe_____

3. Any fluctuations in intracranial pressure? Yes__ No__

SELF-PERCEPTION AND SELF-CONCEPT PATTERN

Subjective

1. What is your major concern at the current time_____

_____

2. Do you think this admission will cause any life style changes for you? No__ Yes__ What_____

3. Do you think this admission will result in any body changes for you? No__ Yes__ What_____

4. My usual view of myself is: Positive__ Neutral__ Somewhat negative __

5. Do you believe you will have any problems dealing with your current health situation? No__ Yes__ Describe_____

6. On a scale of 0-5 rank your perception of your level of control in this situation _____

7. On a scale of 0-5 rank your usual assertiveness level___

8. Have you recently experienced a loss? No__ Yes__ Describe_____

_____

Objective

1. During assessment, patient appears: Calm__ Anxious__ Irritable__ Withdrawn__

   Restless____

2. Did any physiological parameters change: Face reddened? No__ Yes__;

   Voice volume changed? No__ Yes__; Louder__; Softer__;

   Voice quality changed? No__ Yes__; Quavering__; Hesitation__;

   Other_____

3. Body Language Observed_____

4. Is current admission going to result in a body structure or function change

   for the patient? No__ Yes__ Unsure at this time__

ROLE-RELATIONSHIP PATTERN

Subjective

1. Does pt. live alone? Yes__ No__ Who_____

2. Is patient married? Yes__ No__; Children? No__ Yes__; # of children___;

   Age(s) of children_____

   Were any of the children premature? No__ Yes__ Describe_____

   _____

3. How would you rate your parenting skills: Not Applicable__

   No difficulty with__ Average__ Some difficulty with__ Describe_____

4.   Any losses (physical, psychological, social) in past year? No__ Yes__

       Describe_____

5.   How is patient handling this loss at this time_____

       _____

6.   Do you believe this admission will result in any type of loss? No__ Yes__

       Describe_____

7.   Ask both patient and family: Do you think this admission will cause any

       significant changes in (the patient's) usual family role? No__ Yes__

       Describe:_____

8.   How would you rate your usual social activities? Very active__ Active__

       Limited__ None__

9.   How would you rate your comfort in social situations? Comfortable__

       Uncomfortable__

10.   What activities/jobs, etc., do you like to do?_____

       _____

11.   What activities/jobs, etc., do you dislike doing?_____

       _____

12.   Does the person use alcohol or drugs? No__ Yes__ Kind_____

       Amount_____

Objective

1.   Speech Pattern.

       a.   Is English the patient's native language? Yes__ No__

              Native language is_____; Interpreter needed? No__

Yes__

b. During interview have you noted any speech problems? No__ Yes__

Describe_____

2. Family Interaction

a. During interview have you observed any dysfunctional family interactions:

No__ Yes__ Describe_____

b. If patient is child, is there any physical/emotional evidence of physical or

psychosocial abuse? No__ Yes__ Describe_____

_____

c. If patient is a child, is there evidence of attachment behaviors between

parents and child? Yes__ No__ Describe_____

_____

d. Any signs or symptoms of alcoholism? No__ Yes__ Describe_____

_____

SEXUALITY-REPRODUCTIVE PATTERN

Subjective

Female

1. Date of LMP_____; Any pregnancies: Para_____ Gravida_____

Menopause? No__ Yes__ Year_____

2. Use birth control measures? No__ N/A__ Yes__ Type_____

3. Any history of vaginal discharge, bleeding, lesions? No__ Yes__ Discharge

Description_____

4. Pap Smear Annually? Yes__ No__ Date of last Pap Smear_____

5. Date of last Mammogram_____

6.   History of STD (sexually transmitted disease)? No__ Yes__ Describe____

_____

If admission secondary to rape.

7.   Is patient describing numerous physical symptoms? No__ Yes__ Describe

_____

8.   Is patient exhibiting numerous emotional reactions? No__ Yes__ Describe_

_____

9.   What has been your primary coping mechanism to handle this rape episode

_____

10.   Have you talked to persons from the rape crisis center? Yes__ No__

           If no, want you to contact them for her? No__ Yes__

           If yes, was this contact of assistance? No__ Yes__

Male

1.   Any history of prostate problems? No__ Yes__ Describe_____

_____

2.   Any history of penile discharge, bleeding, lesions? No__ Yes__ Describe__

_____

3.   Date of last prostate exam_____

4.   History of STD (sexually transmitted disease)? No__ Yes__

           Describe_____

Both

1.   Are you experiencing any problems in sexual functioning? No__ Yes__

           Describe_____

2.   Are you satisfied with your sexual relationship? Yes__ No__ Describe____

3.   Do you believe this admission will have any impact on sexual functioning?

No___ Yes___ Describe_____

Objective

Review admission physical exam for results of pelvic and rectal exams. If results not

documented nurse should perform exams. Check history to see if admission resulted from a

rape.

COPING-STRESS-TOLERANCE PATTERN

Subjective

1.   Have you experienced any stressful/traumatic events in the past year in addition to

this admission? No__ Yes__ Describe_____

_____

2.   How would you rate your usual handling of stress: Good__ Average__

Poor__

3.   What is the primary way you deal with stress/problems?_____

_____

4.   Have you or your family used any support/counseling groups in the past

year? No__ Yes__ Group Name_____

Was support group helpful? Yes__ No__ Additional comments_____

_____

5.   What do you believe is the primary reason behind the need for this admission?

_____

6.   How soon, after first noting symptoms, did you seek health care assistance?

_____

7. Are you satisfied with the care you have been receiving at home?

   Yes__ No__ Comments_____

8. Ask primary care giver: What is your understanding of the care that will be needed

   when the patient goes home_____

   _____

Objective

1. Observe behavior. Are there any overt signs of stress (e.g., crying, wringing of

   hands, clenched fists, etc.)? Describe_____

   _____

VALUE-BELIEF PATTERN

Subjective

1. Satisfied with the way your life has been developing? Yes__ No__

   Comments_____

2. Will this admission interfere with your plans for the future? No__ Yes__

   How_____

3. Religion: Protestant__ Catholic__ Jewish__ Islam__ Buddhist__

4. Will this admission interfere with your spiritual or religious practices? No__

   Yes__ What_____

5. Any religious restrictions to care (diet, blood transfusions)_____

6. Would you like to have your (pastor, priest, rabbi, hospital chaplain) contacted to

   visit you? No__ Yes__ Which_____

7. Have your religious beliefs helped you to deal with problems in the past?

   No__ Yes___Comments_____

Objective

1. Observe behavior. Is the patient exhibiting any signs of alterations in mood (e.g., anger, crying, withdrawal, etc.)? No__ Yes__ What_____

GENERAL

1. Is there any information we need to have that I have not covered in this interview? No__ Yes__ Comments_____

2. Do you have any questions you need to ask me concerning your health, plan of care or this agency? No__ Yes__ Questions_____

   _____

3. What is the first problem you would like to have assistance with?_____

   _____

MR. FRED CARSON

Mr. Fred Carson is a 63-year-old man who has been admitted with a medical diagnosis of hyperglycemia secondary to diabetes mellitus. He was first diagnosed as having adult onset diabetes 2 years ago.

On admission Mr. Carson's vital signs are: temperature 101.4 degrees F. orally, pulse 98, respiration 20, blood pressure 98/70. Mr. Carson is 5 feet 9 inches tall and weighs 230 pounds. He states he has gained 20 lbs. over the past 6 weeks. His fasting glucose is 200 mg/dL. His hgb. level is 20 g/dL. and an hct. of 56 vol/dL. Mr. Carson tells you he regulates his insulin according to what he eats and eats whatever he is hungry for. You find, in interviewing Mr. Carson, that he has been drinking 3-4 "ice tea glasses" of water every hour stating "I'm always thirsty." He has been voiding at least once an hour. His urine specimen is dilute and a very pale yellow. Mr. Carson's urine glucose, as measure by a clinitest, is 4+. In the past 2 hours Mr. Carson voided 1500 cc's in addition to the urine specimen and his intake has been 500 cc's. Mr. Carson says he doesn't pay any attention to his urine tests, "They're just a waste of time" but, does add "I've been peeing a lot more that past few days. Does this mean I'm not behaving?" Mr. Carson states he was taught about his diabetes but thinks "They were just trying to scare me. I don't think I really have diabetes; kids develop that not old codgers like me. I only check in with the doc when I feel like it. He wants me to come in every other month but, I think he's just trying to get more money." When asked to discuss what he was taught regarding his diabetes Mr. Carson relates a high level of understanding of his prescribed regimen.

You find out this is Mr. Carson's fourth admission over the last 8 months. All of the admissions have been due to complications secondary to the diabetes. He exhibits anger on each admission and refused to have home health nurses visit him.

In examining Mr. Carson's skin you find that his toenails and fingernails are dry, thick, and brittle. Both his skin and mucous membranes are dry in spite of the amount of fluid Mr. Carson indicates he was drinking prior to admission. His extremities are shiny, cool to the touch, and his legs become cyanotic when they are kept in a dependent position. When elevated his legs become pale and color is very slow to return when his legs are returned to a neutral position. His pedal pulses are difficult to locate and diminished in volume. He has a 10 cm.+ size lesion on his left shin and you can see that the lesion has begun to impact the muscle tissue. Mr. Carson tells you he hit his leg on a table 3 weeks ago. You note 3 round scars with atrophied skin on his right leg and 1 similar scar on his left leg. Mr. Carson describes a sensation of "pins and needles when walking but, if I stop it goes away."

ADMISSION ASSESSMENT

DEMOGRAPHIC DATA

Date:_ 10/25/92 _Time:_ 9:25a.m.

Name:_ Carson, Fred

D.O.B.:_ 6/10/29 _____ Age:_ 63 _____ Sex:_ male ____

Primary Significant Other:_ WIFE--RUTH CARSON _____ Telephone #:_ 806-745-5689

Name of Primary Information Source:_ PATIENT

Admitting Medical Diagnosis:_ HYPERGLYCEMIA SECONDARY TO INSULIN

DEPENDENT DIABETES ____

VITAL SIGNS

Temperature_ 101.4 _ F X_ C__ Oral X_ Rectal__ Axillary__ Tympanic__

Pulse Rate: Radial_ 98 _ Apical_____; Regular X_ Irregular__

Respiratory Rate_ 20 _ Abdominal__ Diaphragmatic X_____

Blood Pressure: Left Arm_ 98/60 _; Right Arm_ 100/64 _; Sitting X_ Standing__ Lying

Down__

Weight_ 230 _ pounds, _____kilogram; Height:_ 5 feet 9 inches, _____meters.

Do you have any allergies? No X_ Yes__ What?_____

(Check reactions to medications, foods, cosmetics, insect bites, etc.)

Review admission CBC, Urinalyses, and Chest X-ray. Note any abnormalities here:

FASTING GLUCOSE 200 MG/DL; HGB 20 G/DL; HCT 56 VOL/DL;

HEALTH PERCEPTION/HEALTH MANAGEMENT PATTERN

Subjective

1.   How would you describe your usual health status? Good__ Fair X_ Poor__

40

2. Are you satisfied with your usual health status? Yes__ No X_____

    Source of Dissatisfaction "I'M ALWAYS THIRSTY."_____

3. Tobacco Use? No X Yes__ Number of packs per day_____

4. Alcohol Use? No X Yes__ How much and what kind_____

5. Street Drug Use? No X Yes__ What_____

6. Any history of chronic diseases? No__ Yes X What "THE DOCTOR SAYS I

    HAVE DIABETES, BUT I DON'T BELIEVE IT. KIDS DEVELOP THAT, NO

    OLD CODGERS LIKE ME."_____

7. Immunization History: Tetanus 1960 ; Pneumonia NO ; Influenza NO ;

    MMR HAD DISEASES AS CHILD ; Polio NO ; Hepatitis B NO ; Hib NO

8. Have you sought any health care assistance in the past year? No__ Yes X_____

    If yes, why? "I'M THIRSTY ALL THE TIME." "SORES ON MY LEGS."

    FOUR ADMISSIONS IN PAST 8 MONTHS FOR COMPLICATIONS OF

    DIABETES.____

9. Are you currently working? Yes__ No RETIRED How would you rate your

    working conditions (e.g., safety, noise, space, heating, cooling, water, ventilation)?

    Excellent__ Good__ Fair__ Poor__ Describe any problems areas_____

    _____

10. How would you rate living conditions at home? Excellent X Good__ Fair__

    Poor__ Describe any problem areas "NEED ANOTHER BATHROOM. WE

    HAVE ONLY ONE   AND I NEED TO PEE ALL THE TIME."_____

    _____

11. Do you have any difficulty securing any of the following services?

    Grocery Store? Yes__ No X ; Pharmacy? Yes__ No X ;

Health Care Facility? Yes__ No_X_; Transportation? Yes__ No_X_;

Telephone (for police, fire, ambulance, etc.)? Yes__ No_X_;

If any difficulties, note referral here_____

12. Medications (Over-the-Counter and Prescriptive)

NAME	DOSAGE AMT.	TIMES/DAY	REASON	TAKING AS ORDERED
INSULIN	REGULATES ACCORD.	1-3 TIMES	DIABETES	Yes__ No__
				Yes__ No_
				Yes__ No_
				Yes__ No_
				Yes__ No_
				Yes__ No_
				Yes__ No_
				Yes__ No_

13. Have you followed the routine prescribed for you? Yes__ No_X_____

Why not? "I TAKE THE INSULIN, BUT I DON'T LIKE THE DIET."

14. Did you think this prescribed routine was the best for you? Yes__ No_X_____

What would be better? "I COULD EAT WHAT I WANT."

15. Have you had any accidents/injuries/falls in the past year? No__ Yes_X_____

Describe "I HIT MY LEG ON THE TABLE A FEW WEEKS AGO."

16. Have you had any problems with cuts healing? No__ Yes_X_ Describe "THIS

SORE HAS BEEN HERE SINCE I HIT IT 3 WEEKS AGO (POINTS TO LT

SHIN). THESE SCARS ARE FROM SORES THAT TOOK AGES TO HEAL

(POINTS TO RT LEG)."

42

17. Do you exercise on a regular basis? No _X_ Yes __ Type and Frequency _"I USED TO WALK EVERY AFTERNOON, BUT SINCE I HAVE TO PEE SO MUCH I CAN'T LEAVE THE HOUSE."_

18. Have you experienced any ringing in the ears? Right - Yes __ No _X_

    Left - Yes __ No _X_

19. Have you experienced any vertigo? Yes __ No _X_ How often and when ___

    _____

20. Do you regularly use seat belts? Yes ___ No _X_

21. For infants and children, are car seats used regularly? Yes ___ No ___

22. Do you have any suggestions or assistance requests for improving your health?

    No __ Yes _"I WANT TO STOP PEEING SO MUCH."_

23. Do you do (breast/testicular) self examination? No _X_ Yes __

    How often? _____

24. Were you or your family able to meet all your therapeutic needs? Yes _X_ No __

25. Are you scheduled for surgery? Yes __ No _X_

26. Have you recently had surgery? No _X_ Yes __ Date _____

Objective

1. Mental Status (Indicate assessment with an X)

    a. Oriented _X_ Disoriented __ Length of time _____

       Time: Yes _X_ No __ Length of time _____

       Place: Yes _X_ No __ Length of time _____

       Person: Yes _X_ No __ Length of time _____

    b. Sensorium

Alert__; Drowsy_X_; Lethargic__; Stuporous__; Comatose__;

Cooperative_X_; Combative__; Delusions__; Fluctuating levels of

consciousness? Yes__ No_X_

Appropriate response to stimuli? Yes_X_ No__

    c.   Memory

Recent? Yes_X_ No__; Remote? Yes_X_ No__; Past 4 hours? Yes__ No__

    d.   Is there a disruption of the flow of energy surrounding the person? Yes_X_

No__Change in color? Yes__ No_X_; Change in temperature? Yes__ No

_X_;Field? Yes__ No_X_; Movement? Yes__ No_X_; Sound? Yes__ No_X___

    e.   Responds to simple directions? Yes_X_ No__

2.   Vision

    a.   Visual Acuity: Both eyes 20/___ Right 20/___ Left 20/___ Not assessed

_X_

    b.   Pupil Size: Right - Normal_X_ Abnormal; Left - Normal_X_ Abnormal__

Description of Abnormalities_____

    c.   Pupil Reaction: Right - Normal__ Abnormal__; Left - Normal__

Abnormal__Description of Abnormalities_none_

    d.   Wears Glasses? Yes_X_ No__; Contact Lenses? Yes__ No_X___

3.   Hearing: Not assessed__

    a.   Right - WNL_X_ Impaired__ Deaf__; Left - WNL_X_ Impaired__ Deaf__

    b.   Hearing Aid? Yes__ No_X___

4.   Taste

    a.   Sweet: Normal__ Abnormal__ Describe_NOT EXAMINED_

    b.   Sour: Normal__ Abnormal__ Describe_NOT EXAMINED___

c. Tongue Movement: Normal X Abnormal__ Describe MIDLINE

d. Tongue Appearance: Normal X Abnormal__ Describe PINK, NO LESIONS OR EXUDATE

5. Touch

a. Blunt: Normal X Abnormal__ Describe RESPONDS TO TOUCH ON ALL EXTREMITIES WITH FLAT TONGUE DEPRESSOR

b. Sharp: Normal__ Abnormal X Describe DIMINISHED RESPONSE ON LT FOOT

c. Light Touch Sensation: Normal__ Abnormal X Describe HYPERESTHESIA LT ANKLE AND RT LEG

d. Proprioception: Normal X Abnormal__ Describe

e. Heat: Normal__ Abnormal X Describe DIMINISHED RESPONSE LT FOOT

f. Cold: Normal__ Abnormal X Describe DIMINISHED RESPONSE LT FOOT

g. Any Numbness? No__ Yes X Describe BILATERALLY IN FEET WHEN WALKING

h. Any Tingling? No__ Yes X Describe "PINS AND NEEDLES IN FEET" WHEN WALKING

6. Smell

a. Rt Nostril: Normal X Abnormal__ Describe

b. Lt Nostril: Normal X Abnormal__ Describe

7. Assess Cranial Nerves: Normal X Abnormal___

Describe deviations

45

8. Cerebellar Exam (Romberg, Balance, Gait, Coordination, etc.): Normal__ Abnormal _X_ Describe _ROMBERG ABSENT, BALANCE GOOD, DOES NOT BEAR FULL WEIGHT ON LT FOOT_____

9. Assess Reflexes: Normal _X_ Abnormal_ Describe_____

_____

10. Throat: Enlarged tonsils? No X Yes__ Location _NOT SWOLLEN_____

Tenderness? No _X_ Yes__ Exudate on tonsils? No _X_ Yes__ Color _____

Uvula midline? No__ Yes _X___

11. Neck: Any enlarged lymph nodes? No _X_ Yes__Location and size_____

_____

12. General Appearance

   a.   Hair _BROWN, THINNING_____

   b.   Skin _PALE PINK, DRY, DECREASED TURGOR_____

   c.   Nails_TOENAILS AND FINGERNAILS DRY, THICK, AND

         BRITTLE_____

   d.   Body Odor _NONE_____

NUTRITIONAL/METABOLIC PATTERN

Subjective

1. Any weight gain in last 6 months? No__ Yes _X_ Amount _20 LBS IN LAST 6 WEEKS_____

2. Any weight loss in last 6 months? No _X_ Yes__ Amount_____

3. Would you describe your appetite as: Good _X_ Fair__ Poor__

4. Do you have any food intolerances? No _X_ Yes__ Describe_____

_____

46

5. Do you have any dietary restrictions? (Check for those that are a part of a prescribed regimen as well as those patient restricts voluntarily; e.g., to prevent flatus.)No__ Yes_X_ What "SPECIAL DIET MY WIFE FIXES ME FOR DIABETES."

6. Describe an average day's food intake for you (meals and snacks)

    BREAKFAST: 3 PANCAKES WITH LOW SUGAR SYRUP, JUICE, BLACK COFFEE, SAUSAGE; LUNCH: SANDWICH, MILK OR SUGAR-FREE SOFT DRINK, POTATO CHIPS, FRUIT, "SOMETIMES A LITTLE CAKE OR PIE;" DINNER: CASSEROLE, ICED TEA, ROLLS WITH BUTTER, VEGETABLES AND DESSERT ("SURE DO LIKE MY ICE CREAM"). SNACKS: COOKIES AND JUICE.

7. Describe an average day's fluid intake for you "I DRINK ALL THE TIME," AT LEAST 4 LARGE GLASSES PER HOUR.

8. Describe food likes and dislikes LIKES: MEAT, DESSERTS AND POTATOES   DISLIKES: VEGETABLES, LOW SUGAR "STUFF

9. Would you like to: Gain weight__ Lose weight_X_ Neither__

10. Any problems with:

    a. Nausea? No_X_ Yes__ Describe_____

    b. Vomiting? No_X_ Yes__ Describe_____

    c. Swallowing? No_X_ Yes__ Describe_____

    d. Chewing? No_X_ Yes__ Describe_____

    e. Indigestion? No_X_ Yes__ Describe_____

11. Would you describe your usual lifestyle as: Active__ Sedate_X_

For breastfeeding mothers only:

12. Do you have any concerns about breastfeeding? No___ Yes___

Describe_____

13. Are you having any problems with breastfeeding? No___ Yes___

Describe_____

Objective

1. Skin Examination

   a. Warm___; Cool X ; Moist___; Dry X___

   b. Lesions? No___ Yes X Describe 10 CM+ LT SHIN SEVERAL CM

   DEEP; RED   3 ROUND SCARS WITH ATROPHIED SKIN ON RT

   LEG; 1 ON LT LEG.___

   c. Rash? No X Yes___ Describe_____

   d. Turgor: Firm___; Supple___; Dehydrated X ; Fragile___

   e. Color: Pale___; Pink___; Dusky___; Cyanotic___; Jaundiced___; Mottled___;

   Other PINK EXCEPT FOR LEGS. LEGS ARE CYANOTIC IN

   DEPENDENT POSITION; PALE WHEN ELEVATED._____

   _____

2. Mucous Membranes

   a. Mouth

      (1) Moist___ Dry X___

      (2) Lesions? No X Yes___ Describe_____

      (3) Color: Pale X Pink___

      (4) Teeth: Normal X Abnormal___ Describe_____

      (5) Dentures? No___ Yes___ Upper___ Lower___ Partial X____

      (6) Gums: Normal X Abnormal___ Describe_____

48

        (7)   Tongue: Normal_X_ Abnormal__ Describe_____

  b.   Eyes

        (1)   Moist__ Dry_X_

        (2)   Color of conjunctiva: Pale__ Pink_X_ Jaundiced__

        (3)   Lesions? No_X_ Yes__ Describe_____

5.   Edema

  a.   General? No_X_ Yes__ Describe_____

      _____

      Abdominal Girth _____inches; Not measured _X_____

  b.   Periorbital? No_X_ Yes__

      Describe_____

  c.   Dependent? No__ Yes_X_ Describe BILATERAL ANKLES AND FEET
      WHEN DEPENDENT; LEGS SHINY; NO PITTING.

      Ankle Girth: Right _____inches; Left _____inches; Not

      measured_X_

6.   Thyroid: Normal_X_ Abnormal__ Describe_____

7.   Jugular Vein Distention? No_X_ Yes__

8.   Gag Reflex: Present_X_ Absent__

9.   Can patient move self easily (turning, walking)? Yes__ No_X_____

      Describe limitations DOES NOT BEAR FULL WEIGHT ON LEG; TURNING

      OK.____

10.   Upon admission was patient dressed appropriately for the weather? Yes_X_

      No___Describe_____

For Breastfeeding Mothers Only

11. Breast Exam: Normal__ Abnormal__ Describe_____

_____

12. Weigh infant. Is infant's weight within normal limits? Yes__ No__

ELIMINATION PATTERN

Subjective

1. What is your usual frequency of bowel movements? <u>ABOUT 3 TIMES</u>

    <u>PER WEEK.</u>

    a. Have to strain to have BM? No_X_ Yes__

    b. Same time each day? No_X_ Yes__

2. Has the number of bowel movements changed in the past week? No_X_

    Yes__Increased__ Decreased__

3. Character of stool:

    a. Consistency: Hard__ Soft_X_ Liquid__

    b. Color: Brown_X_ Black__ Yellow__ Clay colored__

    c. Bleeding with bowel movements? No__ Yes__

4. History of constipation? No_X_ Yes__ How often_____

    Use bowel movement aids (laxatives, suppositories, diet)? No_X_ Yes__

    Describe_____

5. History of diarrhea? No_X_ Yes__ When_____

6. History of Incontinence? No_X_ Yes__

    Related to increased abdominal pressure (coughing, laughing, sneezing)? No__

    Yes__

7. History of recent travel? No_X_ Yes__ Where_____

8. Usual voiding pattern:

a. Frequency (times/day) FOR PAST 3 DAYS, 3-4/HOUR Decreased__ Increased X____

b. Change in Awareness of Need to Void? No__ Yes X____ Increased__ Decreased X____

c. Change in Urge to Void? No__ Yes X Increased X Decreased__

b. Any Change in Amount? No__ Yes X Decreased__ Increased X____

c. Color: Yellow VERY PALE Smokey__ Dark__

d. Incontinence? No__ Yes X When "IF TOO FAR FROM BATHROOM."
_____

Difficulty holding voiding when urge to void develops? No__ Yes X

Have time to get to bathroom? Yes__ No X____

How often does problem reaching bathroom occur EVERY VOIDING
_____

e. Retention? No X Yes__ Describe_____

f. Pain/burning? No X Yes__ Describe_____

g. Sensation of bladder spasms? No X Yes__ When_____

Objective

1. Auscultate abdomen.

   a. Bowel Sounds: Normal X Increased__ Decreased__ Absent__

2. Palpate abdomen.

   a. Tender? No X Yes__ Where?_____

   b. Soft? Yes X No__; Firm? Yes__ No X____

   c. Masses? No X Yes__ Describe_____

d.   Distention (include distended bladder)? No X Yes__ Describe____

_____

e.   Overflow urine when bladder palpated? Yes__ No X____

3.   Rectal Exam

a.   Sphincter tone: Describe WITHIN NORMAL LIMITS_____

b.   Hemorrhoids? No X Yes__ Describe_____

c.   Stool in rectum? No__ Yes X Describe HEME NEGATIVE____

d.   Impaction? No X Yes__ Describe_____

e.   Occult Blood? No X Yes__

4.   Ostomy Present? No X Yes__ Location_____

ACTIVITY-EXERCISE PATTERN

Subjective

1.   Using the Functional Level Classification below have patient rate each area of self

care. (Code adapted by NANDA from E. Jones, et al. Patient Classification for

Long-Term care: Users' Manual, HEW, Publication No. HRA-74-3107.

November, 1974).

        0 = Completely independent

        1 = Requires use of equipment or device.

        2 = Requires help from another person, for assistance, supervision,

            or teaching.

        3 = Requires help from another person and equipment device.

        4 = Dependent, does not participate in activity.

Feeding 0 ; Bathing/Hygiene 0 ; Dressing/Grooming 0 ;

Toileting 0 ; Ambulation 0 ; Care of home WIFE ; Shopping WIFE ;

52

Meal preparation WIFE ; Laundry WIFE ; Transportation   0   .

2.   Oxygen use at home? No X Yes__ Describe_____

3.   How many pillows do you use to sleep on: Number 1_____

4.   Do you frequently experience fatigue? No__ Yes X Describe "I'M TIRED

AFTER GOING TO THE BATHROOM SO MUCH."_____

5.   How many stairs can you climb without experiencing any difficulty?

Number (can be individual number or number of flights) 1 FLIGHT_____

6.   How far can you walk without experiencing any difficulty? 1 BLOCK; "MY

FOOT HURTS IF I TRY TO WALK TOO FAR."_____

7.   Has assistance at home for care of self and maintenance of home? No__ Yes X

Who WIFE_____

If No, would like to have or believes needs to have assistance? No__ Yes__ With

What Activities_____

8.   Occupation (if retired, former occupation) MAIL CARRIER_____

9.   Describe your usual leisure time activities/hobbies GARDENING,

FISHING, READING

10.   Any complaints of weakness or lack of energy? No__ Yes X_____

Describe GOING TO THE BATHROOM SO MUCH "WEARS ME OUT."_____

_____

11.   Any difficulties in maintaining activities of daily living? No__ Yes X_____

Describe "ALL I DO IS DRINK AND PEE."_____

12.   Any problems with concentration? No X Yes__ Describe_____

_____

Objective

53

1. Cardiovascular

    a.   Cyanosis? No__ Yes _X_ Where LEGS WHEN DEPENDENT

    b.   Pulses: Easily palpable?

              Carotid--Yes _X_ No__; Jugular--Yes _X_ No__; Temporal--Yes _X_ No__;

              Radial--Yes _X_ No__; Femoral--Yes _X_ No__; Popliteal--Yes _X_ No__;

              Post Tibial--Yes__ No _X_ ; Dorsalis pedis--Yes__ No _X_

    c. Extremities:

          (1)   Temperature: Cold__ Cool _X_ Warm__ Hot__

          (2)   Capillary Refill: Normal__ Delayed _X_

          (3)   Color: Pink__ Pale _X_ Cyanotic _X_ Other__

                  Describe PALE WHEN RAISED; CYANOTIC WHEN

                  DEPENDENT

          (4)   Homan's Sign? No _X_ Yes__

              (5)   Nails: Normal__ Abnormal _X_ Describe TOENAILS

                      AND FINGER-NAILS DRY, THICK, BRITTLE

              (6)   Hair Distribution: Normal _X_ Abnormal__

                      Describe____

              (7)   Claudication? No__ Yes _X_ Describe NUMBNESS AND

                      TINGLING IN FEET

    d.   Heart: PMI Location 4TH ICS LCL

          (1)   Abnormal rhythm? No _X_ Yes__ Describe____

          (2)   Abnormal sounds? No _X_ Yes__ Describe____

2. Respiratory

    a.   Rate _20/MIN__ ; Depth - Shallow__ Deep_X_ Abdominal__ Diaphragmatic

        X

    b.   Have patient cough. Any sputum? No _X_ Yes__ Describe_____

        _____

    c.   Fremitus? No _X_ Yes__

    d.   Any chest excursion? No _X_ Yes__ Equal__ Unequal__

    e.   Ausculatate Chest:

        Any abnormal sounds (Rales, Rhonchi)? No _X_ Yes__Describe___

        _____

    f.   Have pt. walk in place for 3 minutes (if permissible):

        (1)   Any shortness of breath after activity? No _X_ Yes__

        (2)   Any dyspnea? No _X_ Yes__

        (3)   B.P. after activity_ 108 _/_ 74 _ in (Rt; Left) arm.

        (4)   Respiratory rate after activity__ 25 _____

        (5)   Pulse rate after activity_ 110 ____

3. Musculo-Skeletal

    a.   Range of motion: Normal__ Limited_X_ Describe LIMITED IN LOWER

        EXTREMITIES_____

    b.   Gait: Normal__ Abnormal_X_ Describe DOES NOT BEAR FULL

        WEIGHT ON__ LEFT ANKLE_____

    c.   Balance: Normal_X_ Abnormal__ Describe_____

    d.   Muscle Mass/Strength: Normal__ Increased__ Decreased _X_____

Describe ATROPHY IN BOTH LEGS, ESPECIALLY IN AREA OF

WOUNDS

    e.   Hand Grasp: Right - Normal X Decreased__

             Left - Normal X Decreased__

    f.   Toe Wiggle: Right - Normal X Decreased__

             Left - Normal X Decreased__

    g.   Posture: Normal X Kyphosis__ Lordosis__

    h.   Deformities? No X Yes__ Describe_____

    i.   Missing limbs? No X Yes__ Where_____

    j.   Uses mobility assistive devices (walker, crutches, etc.)? No X

             Yes__ Describe_____

    k.   Tremors? No X Yes__ Describe_____

    l.   Traction or Casts present? No X Yes__ Describe_____

4.   Spinal Cord Injury? No X Yes__ Level_____

5.   Paralysis present? No X Yes__ Where_____

6.   Conduct developmental assessment. Normal__ Abnormal__ Describe NOT

DONE

7.   Responds appropriately to stimuli? Yes X No__ Describe_____

8.   Are there any abnormal movements? No X Yes__ Describe_____

SLEEP-REST PATTERN

Subjective

1.   Usual sleep habits: Hours/night__6__; Naps? No__ Yes X AM__ PM X

Feel rested? Yes _X_ No __ Describe_____

2.   Any problems:

     a.   Difficulty going to sleep? No _X_ Yes __

     b.   Awakening during night? No __ Yes _X (TO GO TO THE BATHROOM)_

     c.   Early awakening? No _X_ Yes __

     d.   Insomnia? No _X_ Yes __ Describe_____

3.   Methods used to promote sleep: Medication? No _X_ Yes __ Name_____

_____

Warm fluids? No _X_ Yes __ What_____

Relaxation techniques? No _X_ Yes __

Objective

None

COGNITIVE-PERCEPTUAL PATTERN

Subjective

1.　Pain.

    a.　Location (have pt. point to)　LEFT SHIN

    b.　Intensity (have pt. rank on scale of 0-10)　5

    c.　Radiation? No__ Yes X To where UP LEG

    d.　Timing (how often; related to any specific events) "ACHES ALL THE TIME;"

        INCREASED PAIN WITH WALKING OR IF TOUCH WOUND.

    e.　Duration AS ABOVE

    f.　What do to relieve at home ELEVATE, TAKE AN ADVIL

    g.　When did pain begin "TWO WEEKS AGO"

2.　Decision Making

    a.　Find decision making: Easy X Moderately easy__ Moderately difficult__ Difficult__

    b.　Inclined to make decisions: Rapidly X Slowly__ Delay__

    c.　Difficulty choosing between options? Yes__ No X

        Describe

3.　Knowledge level

    a.　Can define what current problem is? Yes X No__

    b.　Can restate current therapeutic regimen? Yes X No__

Objective

1. Review sensory and mental status completed in Health Perception-Health

   Management Pattern.

2. Any overt signs of pain? No__ Yes _X_ Describe WINCES WHEN TRIES TO

   BEAR WEIGHT ON LEFT LEG

3. Any fluctuations in intracranial pressure? Yes__ No__

SELF-PERCEPTION AND SELF-CONCEPT PATTERN

Subjective

1. What is your major concern at the current time _"I'M TIRED OF DOING_

   NOTHING BUT DRINKING AND PEEING."

2. Do you think this admission will cause any life style changes for you? No__ Yes

   _X_ What _"HELP ME GET BETTER"_

3. Do you think this admission will result in any body changes for you? No__ Yes _X_

   _____What _"HEAL MY LEG."_

4. My usual view of myself is: Positive _X_ Neutral__ Somewhat negative __

5. Do you believe you will have any problems dealing with your current health

   situation? No _X_ Yes__ Describe

6. On a scale of 0-5 rank your perception of your level of control in this   situation

   _4_

7. On a scale of 0-5 rank your usual assertiveness level _5_

8. Have you recently experienced a loss? No _X_ Yes__ Describe

Objective

1. During assessment, patient appears: Calm__ Anxious__ Irritable X Withdrawn__

   Restless____

2. Did any physiological parameters change: Face reddened? No X Yes__;

   Voice volume changed? No X Yes__; Louder__; Softer__;

   Voice quality changed? No X Yes__; Quavering__; Hesitation__;

   Other_____

3. Body Language Observed GUARDS LEFT SHIN_____

4. Is current admission going to result in a body structure or function change for the

   patient? No__ Yes__ Unsure at this time X_____

ROLE-RELATIONSHIP PATTERN

Subjective

1. Does pt. live alone? Yes__ No X Who WIFE_____

2. Is patient married? Yes X No__; Children? No X Yes__; # of children_____;

   Age(s) of children_____

   Were any of the children premature? No__ Yes__ Describe N/A_____

   _____

3. How would you rate your parenting skills: Not Applicable X_____

   No difficulty with__ Average__ Some difficulty with__

   Describe_____

4. Any losses (physical, psychological, social) in past year? No__ Yes X_____

   Describe EARLY RETIREMENT_____

5. How is patient handling this loss at this time "DOING FINE, JUST NEED TO

   GET FEET IN SHAPE SO I CAN DO WHAT I WANT NOW THAT I HAVE

   THE TIME."___

6. Do you believe this admission will result in any type of loss? No X Yes__

Describe_____

7. Ask both patient and family: Do you think this admission will cause any significant changes in (the patient's) usual family role? No X Yes__

Describe:_____

8. How would you rate your usual social activities? Very active__ Active X Limited__ None__

9. How would you rate your comfort in social situations? Comfortable X Uncomfortable__

10. What activities/jobs, etc., do you like to do? GARDENING, FISHING, PLAYING CARDS AND DOMINOES_____

11. What activities/jobs, etc., do you dislike doing? ANY HOUSEWORK OR COOKING OR HAVING TO PEE ALL THE TIME_____

12. Does the person use alcohol or drugs? No X Yes__ Kind_____

Amount_____

Objective

1. Speech Pattern.

   a. Is English the patient's native language? Yes X No__

   Native language is_____; Interpreter needed?

   No___Yes__

   b. During interview have you noted any speech problems? No X

   Yes__Describe_____

2. Family Interaction

   a. During interview have you observed any dysfunctional family interactions:

No _X_ Yes __ Describe_____

b. If patient is child, is there any physical/emotional evidence of physical or psychosocial abuse? No__ Yes__Describe___

_____

c. If patient is a child, is there evidence of attachment behaviors between parents and child? Yes__ No__ Describe _N/A_____

_____

d. Any signs or symptoms of alcoholism? No _X_ Yes__

Describe_____

SEXUALITY-REPRODUCTIVE PATTERN

Subjective

Female

1. Date of LMP_____; Any pregnancies: Para_____ Gravida_____
    Menopause? No__ Yes__ Year_____

2. Use birth control measures? No__ N/A__ Yes__ Type_____

3. Any history of vaginal discharge, bleeding, lesions? No__ Yes__
    Discharge_____

4. Pap Smear Annually? Yes__ No__ Date of last Pap Smear_____

5. Date of last Mammogram_____

6. History of STD (sexually transmitted disease)? No__ Yes__ Describe____

_____

If admission secondary to rape.

7. Is patient describing numerous physical symptoms? No__ Yes__ Describe

_____

8.   Is patient exhibiting numerous emotional reactions? No__ Yes__ Describe_

_____

9.   What has been your primary coping mechanism to handle this rape

episode?_____

10.   Have you talked to persons from the rape crisis center? Yes__ No__

If no, want you to contact them for her? No__ Yes__

If yes, was this contact of assistance? No__ Yes__

Male

1.   Any history of prostate problems? No _X_ Yes__ Describe_____

_____

2.   Any history of penile discharge, bleeding, lesions? No _X_ Yes__ Describe_

_____

3.   Date of last prostate exam LAST ADMISSION_____

4.   History of STD (sexually transmitted disease)? No _X_ Yes__ Describe____

_____

Both

1.   Are you experiencing any problems in sexual functioning? No__ Yes _X_____

Describe IMPOTENCY FOR PAST SEVERAL MONTHS_____

2.   Are you satisfied with your sexual relationship? Yes__ No _X_ Describe

IMPOTENT_____

3.   Do you believe this admission will have any impact on sexual functioning? No__

Yes _X_

Describe "GET MY DIABETES UNDER CONTROL AND PROBLEM WILL

BE HELPED."_____

Objective

Review admission physical exam for results of pelvic and rectal exams. If results not documented nurse should perform exams. Check history to see if admission resulted from a rape.

COPING-STRESS-TOLERANCE PATTERN

Subjective

1. Have you experienced any stressful/traumatic events in the past year in addition to this admission? No__ Yes X Describe NUMEROUS ADMISSIONS AND I MISS WORK SOME_____.

2. How would you rate your usual handling of stress: Good__ Average X Poor__

3. What is the primary way you deal with stress/problems YELL OR AVOID SITUATION. "I DON'T LIKE TO TALK ABOUT IT."

4. Have you or your family used any support/counseling groups in the past year? No X Yes__ Group Name_____

    Was support group helpful? Yes__ No__ Additional comments_____

    _____

5. What do you believe is the primary reason behind the need for this admission? "TO GET MY DIABETES UNDER CONTROL AGAIN; I GUESS I'M A SLOW LEARNER."

6. How soon, after first noting symptoms, did you seek health care assistance? 3 WEEKS

7. Are you satisfied with the care you have been receiving at home? Yes X No__ Comments "MY WIFE HAS ALWAYS TAKEN GOOD CARE OF ME

AND I DIDN'T WANT TO HAVE THOSE PEOPLE (V.N.A.) COMING TO

MY HOUSE."

8.   Ask primary care giver: What is your understanding of the care that will be needed

when the patient goes home WIFE NOT PRESENT AT THIS TIME

_____

Objective

1.   Observe behavior. Are there any overt signs of stress (e.g., crying, wringing of

hands, clenched fists, etc.)? Describe CLENCHED FISTS

_____

VALUE-BELIEF PATTERN

Subjective

1.   Satisfied with the way your life has been developing? Yes__ No X_____

Comments "WAS O.K. UNTIL THIS DIABETES DEVELOPED."

2.   Will this admission interfere with your plans for the future? No X Yes__

How_____

3.   Religion: Protestant X Catholic__ Jewish__ Islam__ Buddhist__

4.   Will this admission interfere with your spiritual or religious practices?

No X Yes__ What_____

5.   Any religious restrictions to care (diet, blood transfusions) NO_____

6.   Would you like to have your (pastor, priest, rabbi, hospital chaplain) contacted to

visit you? No X Yes__ Which_____

7.   Have your religious beliefs helped you to deal with problems in the past? No__

Yes X Comments NONE_____

Objective

1. Observe behavior. Is the patient exhibiting any signs of alterations in mood (e.g., anger, crying, withdrawal, etc.)? No__ Yes X What CLENCHED FISTS

    _____

GENERAL

1. Is there any information we need to have that I have not covered in this interview?

    No X Yes__ Comments_____

2. Do you have any questions you need to ask me concerning your health, plan of care or this agency? No X Yes__ Questions_____

    _____

3. What is the first problem you would like to have assistance with? STOP ME FROM HAVING TO GO TO THE BATHROOM ALL THE TIME

PART V–DEVELOPING EXPECTED OUTCOMES

A PROGRAMMED UNIT OF STUDY

BY

HELEN C. COX, R.N., C., Ed.D., F.A.A.N.

TEXAS TECH UNIVERSITY HEALTH SCIENCES CENTER

SCHOOL OF NURSING

LUBBOCK, TEXAS

EXPECTED OUTCOMES

As a result of completing this programmed unit on patient care expected outcomes, the student should be able to:

1. List at least 4 criteria for useful patient care expected outcomes.

2. Write a useful patient care expected outcome.

3. Distinguish between a poorly stated patient care expected outcome and a well stated patient care expected outcome.

4. Identify two reasons for establishing deadlines on patient care expected outcomes.

INTRODUCTION

The third major step in the nursing process is the planning phase. This phase consists of two parts.

Part 1 of the planning phase focuses on establishing patient care expected outcomes. Part 2 of the planning phase consists of setting deadlines for meeting the expected outcomes.

PATIENT CARE EXPECTED OUTCOMES

Briefly defined, patient care expected outcomes "are the day to day levels of performance which the patient must reach in order to eventually attain his long-range goals."

Criteria for useful patient care expected outcomes are:

1. Clearly stated in terms of patient behavior or clinical manifestations.

   EX: Poor--Control of diarrhea.

   Good--Decrease in number of stools to one daily.

   Stools of normal consistency.

2. Realistic--Based on everything known about the patient, achievable and safe.

   EX: Mr. Adams is a 56-year-old man who can briefly be described as a sedentary patient with heart disease.

   One overall goal for Mr. Adams is to increase his exercise tolerance.

   Unrealistic: Jog for 1 mile the first morning of the exercise program.

   Realistic: a. Walk 1 full block every morning of the first week of the exercise program without out dyspnea.

    b. Walk 2 full blocks every morning of the second week

of the exercise program without dyspnea.

3. Acceptable to the patient and his family or significant others.

    EX: Mrs. Braxton is a 28 year old woman who has delayed healing of a   surgical wound. The physician has ordered discharge instructions regarding a high protein diet. Mrs. Braxton is a widow with 3 children below the age of 10. Her only source of income is from social security.

    Unacceptable: Will eat at least one 8 ounce serving of steak   each day.

    Acceptable: Will eat at least one serving of one of the following   each day: Lean ground meat, eggs, cheese, pinto beans, peanut butter.

4. Written in terms depicting patient action,

    EX: Poor--Maintains oral hygiene.

    Good--Brushes teeth and gums after each meal.

5. Specific and concrete.

    EX: Poor--Increases amount of exercise.

    Good--Participates in exercise session at 9:30 a.m. each day.

6. Directly observable by use of at least one of the five senses.

    EX: Poor--Decreased pain.

Good--Decrease in number of complaints about pain.

7. Patient centered rather than nurse centered.

    EX: Poor--Offer urinal or assists to bathroom upon patient's stated need to void.

    Good--Obtains urinal or requests help to bathroom upon need to void.

SETTING DEADLINES

Deadlines serve to facilitate the nursing process in several ways. Establishing deadlines serve to:

1. Pace the patient's nursing care program by helping to keep the patient's progress on target.

2. Motivates both the patient and nurse to strive toward goals. Deadlines endow patient care activities with a sense of purpose and urgency.

3. Provide the patient and staff with a sense of accomplishment when the deadlines are met.

4. Act as a "red flag" when not met; thus, signaling a need to reassess and replan.

Deadlines can be realistically established by reviewing the following:

1. The typical course of the patient's problem and the speed with which problems related symptoms are usually controlled.

2. Resources, capabilities and energy levels of the patient and staff.

3. The patient's own inner time clock and rhythms.

You are now beginning the programmed phase of the unit. Read the situation, choose one

answer then turn to the page number indicated by your chosen answer.

Mr. Adams was admitted to the clinical unit with a medical diagnosis of decubitus ulcer
and the possible need for a skin graft. After the admission assessment the nurse makes the
following nursing diagnosis: Risk for infection secondary to decubitus ulcer.

Which of the following is the most appropriate expected outcome for Mr. Adams?

Mr. Adams:

1. Will not have an increase in the size of the ulcer from 7cm by
   3/7. (See page 86).
2. Will maintain current status by 3/7. (See page 90).
3. Will exhibit no signs or symptoms of infection by 3/7. (See
   page 85)

Yes. This is the best patient care expected outcome. It is clearly stated in terms of what Mr. Cannon will have to do (drink 8 ounces of fluid). It is realistic because Mr. Cannon has no nausea or vomiting and it allows 2 days before time for evaluation. It has a high probability of being acceptable if Mr. Cannon is allowed to select which kind of fluid (juice, water, soft drink, tea, coffee, etc.). It is specific and measurable. Please continue with the program.

Mrs. Dodge is admitted to the hospital on 10/21 with a medical diagnosis of a fractured left tibia and fibula. Mrs. Dodge is 5 feet 4 inches tall and weights 206 pounds. the physician leaves an order for a 900 calorie reducing diet. The admission nurse writes the following nursing diagnosis: Altered Nutrition: More than Body Requirements due to stated lack of knowledge regarding dietary intake, calories, and exercise. Which of the following is the most correct patient care expected outcome for this nursing diagnosis?

Mrs. Dodge will:

1. Select a 900 calorie diet from a dietary exchange list. (See   page 84).

2. Lose three pounds by 10/28. (See page 89).

3. Weigh 15 pounds less by 10/28. (See page 92).

This answer is a tricky one. The content, behavior, etc. is correct; but, there is no deadline date. Return to page 83 and try again.

Good! This is the most correct expected outcome for the stated nursing diagnosis. It meets the stated criteria well. Please proceed with the program.

Mr. Gist is a 24-year-old man who is admitted to the unit on 9/30 following an emergency appendectomy. Mr. Gist is restless, alert and complaining of pain at the incision site. The nurse writes the following diagnosis: Pain secondary to surgical incision. Which of the following is the best expected outcome for this nursing diagnosis?

1. Will give medication as necessary for pain by 10/1. (See page 87).

2. Will request pain medication no more than once per day by   10/3.   (See page 93).

3. Will verbalize ways he can control his pain. (See page 106).

No. This expected outcome does not related to the diagnosis of risk for infection. The ulcer could increase in size (although hopefully we are doing enough good care so it doesn't) without infection being present. Go back to page 82 and try again.

Sorry. This expected outcome is stated in terms of nurse behavior not patient behavior. Return to page 85 and try again.

No. While a reasonably balanced I and O is a goal for each patient, this goal is unrealistic due both to the target date (the majority of patients have a balanced I and O only every 48-72 hours) and the fact that Mr. Cannon has a deficit. We want his intake to exceed his output until the deficit is corrected. Return to page 100 and try again.

Yes. This is the best expected outcome. It is clear, realistic and measurable. Proceed with the program.

Mr. Erwin, a 52-year-old man, is admitted on 1/4 with the medical diagnosis of bilateral lower lobar pneumonia. During the admission assessment, the nurse finds that Mr. Erwin cannot walk more than 50 feet or climb one flight of stairs without stopping. The nurse records the following nursing diagnosis: Decreased Activity Tolerance (Level III) secondary to ineffective airway clearance. Which of the following is the <u>most</u> correct patient care expected outcome for Mr. Erwin?

Mr. Erwin:

1. Will have increased activity tolerance by 1/11. (See page 95).

2. Will accept bed rest restrictions until pneumonia begins to clear (1/11). (See page 98).

3. a. Will ambulate from bed to nurse's station (500 feet) by 1/7 without stopping.

   b. Will ambulate unrestricted distance without respiratory or energy problems by 1/14. (See page 103).

Sorry. Remember the expected outcome has to be specific and measurable. What directions for care does "maintain current status" give? How can you measure "maintain current status"? Return to page 82 and try again.

Sorry. This expected outcome is specific to the medical diagnosis (Empyema) but not the nursing diagnosis. We have to have something in the expected outcome that directly relates to the airway clearance. Return to page 103 and try again.

The only problem with this expected outcome is the realism. While it is possible that someone that weighs as much as Mrs. Dodge does could lose 15 pounds in one week, under close supervision, it is not as realistic as another objective given. We must be cautious so that the expected outcomes show progress not the reverse. What would happen to Mrs. Dodge's attitude and morale if she did not reach this goal? Return to page 83 and try again.

Good. This expected outcome is realistic (3 days postop,), specific, and measurable. Please continue with the program.

Mrs. Hodge is a 43-year-old woman who is admitted to the hospital and is scheduled to have an abdominal hysterectomy on May 3rd (2 days after admission). Mrs. Hodge has been admitted early for a total physical exam (possibility of a malignancy) and to receive blood transfusions prior to surgery (Hgb. of 6.4). Mrs. Hodge has been in the hospital only one time before and that was for the birth of her child. Mrs. Hodge expresses anxiety about her hospitalization, the surgery and the possibility of cancer. The admission nurse records the following nursing diagnosis: Fear secondary to lack of knowledge regarding hospitalization, surgery and diagnosis. Which of the following expected outcomes is the best for this nursing diagnosis?

1. Will verbalize acceptance of the need for surgery by 5/3. (See page 96).

2. Will verbalize understanding of hospital routine, need for surgery and her diagnosis by 5/5. (See page 101).

3 Will freely ask questions regarding hospital routine, her scheduled surgery and her possible diagnosis by 5/2. (See page 104).

Good. This is the most appropriate expected outcome. Signs and symptoms of infection can be observed and measured (heat, swelling, redness, drainage, changes in vital signs, changes in white blood cell counts). Also specifically stating infection gives directions for nursing orders (cleanliness, close observation, protection, turning, etc.). Continue the program by reading the following situation.

Mrs. Baker is a 40-year-old woman admitted on 11/29 with a medical diagnosis of diabetes mellitus. This is her third admission in 8 weeks. Mrs. Baker has been regulating her insulin according to what she eats rather than her urine tests. After the admission assessment, the nurse writes the following nursing diagnosis: Ineffective Management of Therapeutic Regimen (Individual) secondary to stated lack of knowledge regarding urine testing. Which of the following is the <u>most</u> appropriate expected outcome for Mrs. Baker's nursing diagnosis?

1. Will understand the correlation between her urine tests and insulin dose by 12/1. (See page 97).

2. a. Will correctly perform clinitest and acetest by 11/30.

   b. Will correctly measure and self inject insulin based on results of clinitest and acetest by 11/30. (See page 105).

3. a. Will return demonstrate urine testing with 100% accuracy by 12/1.

   b. Will self administer insulin with 100% accuracy with dosage based on urine tests by 12/2. (See page 100).

Not this expected outcome. This expected outcome is nonspecific and unmeasurable. Please return to page 89 and try again.

No. This expected outcome leaves out the other fear related factors so it is not concrete enough. Return to page 93 and try again.

Well, we do, certainly, want her to understand the relationship between what her urine test shows and the amount of insulin she takes; but, how do we measure understanding? Also how realistic is it to expect her to reach the entire goal in two days? Please return to page 94 and try again.

No. Bedrest restrictions and acceptance of these will not help Mr. Erwin's activity tolerance and could increase the pneumonia problem; therefore, this is an unrealistic expected outcome. Return to page 89 and try again.

No. There is a better expected outcome. Mrs. Franklin could verbalize reasons but still not turn, cough, or deep breathe. We do want her to demonstrate understanding of why she is turning, coughing, and deep breathing but it's more important that she actually perform the activities. Return to page 103 and try again.

Great! This is correct. The expected outcomes are specific, clearly stated in terms of patient behavior and action, realistic, and specific. Please continue the program.

Mr. Cannon was admitted on 2/14 with a medical diagnosis of diarrhea due to salmonella. Mr. Cannon has had diarrhea for four days. He has decreased urine output, no nausea or vomiting, has lost 15 pounds in 4 days, has increased temperature and pulse rate, dry skin, decreased skin turgor and complains of weakness. The admission nurse writes the following nursing diagnosis: Fluid Volume Deficit secondary to diarrhea. Which is the following is the most appropriate expected outcome for Mr. Cannon?

1. Will drink at least 8 ounces of fluid every hour from 7 a.m. to 11 p.m. by 12/16. (See page 83).

2. Will have a balanced intake and output by 2/15. (See page 88).

3. Will maintain an I.V. intake of 500 mL each 8 hours by 2/17. (See page 102).

Sorry. Even though this expected outcome meets most of the criteria, the deadline date is 2 days after the scheduled surgery. Please return to page 93 and try again.

Sorry. This expected outcome is stated in terms of nurse behavior. How could Mr. Cannon assure this for himself? In addition, it is probably unrealistic in terms of the amount of fluid replacement Mr. Cannon needs. Please turn back to page 100 and try again.

Yes! This expected outcome is realistic (note the varying dates and length of ambulation), specific, concrete, measurable, and has a high probability of acceptance due to the sequencing of the expected outcomes. The sequencing reinforces progress for both the patient and the nurse. Please proceed with the program.

Mrs. Franklin is a 32-year-old woman admitted 4/22 with a medical diagnosis of empyema. She is having dyspnea and is coughing up small amounts of purulent material. Her temperature is 102 degrees orally, pulse 86, respiration 22 and shallow, and B.P. 138/88. The admitting nurse records the following nursing diagnosis: Ineffective airway clearance related to empyema. Which of the following expected outcomes is the best for this nursing diagnosis?

Mrs. Franklin:

1. Will cough, turn and deep breathe every hour from 8 a.m. to 10 p.m. by 4/23. (See page 85).

2. Will have decreased signs and symptoms of infection (lower T., P., R, B.P.) by 4/27. (See page 91).

3. Will verbalize reasons for coughing, turning, and deep breathing every 2 hours by 4/23. (See page 99).

Good! This is the best expected outcome. It gives direction for nursing intervention, is concrete and specific, is realistic, is clearly stated in terms of patient behavior, will be acceptable because it does not require undue energy and will assist in relieving fear and is measurable.

You have now completed the program. Please turn to page 107 and complete the self evaluation. The answers to the self evaluation immediately follows the self evaluation page.

This answer is certainly better than number 1 but please note that the expected outcomes are not specific. Do we mean demonstrate correctly? Do we mean administer the correct dose correctly? Are we going to include basing the insulin dose on the results of the urine test rather than what she eats? How realistic is it to expect her to do all of this within one day of admission? Please return to page 94 and try again.

No. Patients can help control their pain by using distraction, turning, etc. but the key point is there is no deadline date. Return to page 85 and try again.

SELF EVALUATION

1. List at least four, of the seven, criteria necessary for useful patient care expected outcomes.

1.

2.

3.

4.

2. Mr. Williams is admitted with a medical diagnosis of bilateral phlebitis. During the admission assessment the nurse discovers Mr. Williams has been delaying having bowel movements due to the pain of ambulation. Before this health problem arose Mr. Williams' normal bowel pattern was one stool every a.m. The following nursing diagnosis was made:

Constipation due to difficulty and pain in ambulating to B.R. Write an appropriate nursing care expected outcome for Mr. Williams.

3. For each of the following expected outcomes, and without referring to any earlier part of this program, evaluate each expected outcomes as to being poor or good. If the expected outcome is poor, place a P in front of the expected outcome. If the expected outcome is good, place a G in front of the expected outcome.

_____a. Decrease in number of stools to once daily. Stools of normal

consistency.

_____b. Jog for 1 mile within 1 week of beginning the exercise program.

_____c. Maintain correct oral hygiene.

_____d. Brushes teeth and gums after each meal.

_____e. Increases amount of fluid intake.

_____f. Understands rationale for diet restriction.

_____g. Drinks at least 8 oz. of fluid every awake hour.

_____h. Control of diarrhea.

_____i. Walk one full block every morning of the first week of the exercise program without dyspnea.

_____j. Selects diet from diet exchange table and stays within 900 calories per day.

4. Which of the following are reasons for establishing deadline dates for patient care expected outcomes?

_____a. Documents use of expected outcomes for patient care.

_____b. Acts as a "red flag" when not met; thus, signaling a need to reassess and replan.

_____c. Meets criteria established by JACHO.

_____d. Motivates both patients and nurses to strive toward the goal.

SELF EVALUATION ANSWERS

1. a. Clearly stated in terms of patient behavior or clinical manifestations.

   b. Realistic.

   c. Acceptable to patient and his significant others.

   d. Written in terms depicting patient action.

   e. Specific and concrete.

   f. Directly observable by use of at least one of the 5 senses.

   g. Patient centered rather than nurse centered.

2. Something similar to:

   Mr. Williams will have at least one bowel movement of normal consistency every morning by <u>date</u>.

3. a. G

   b. P (unrealistic)

   c. P (not specific; unmeasurable)

   d. G

   e. P (unspecific, unmeasurable)

   f. P (too general)

   g. G

   h. P (unspecific, etc.)

   i. G

j. G

4. Correct answers are b and d.

CASE STUDY 1

CHRIS APPLETON

Chris Appleton is a 5 year old boy who was admitted this morning with a medical diagnosis of acute lymphocytic leukemia. Chris was originally diagnosed as having leukemia 3 months ago and has been on I.V. chemotherapy since that time. His preschool inoculations have been delayed due to the medical diagnosis and the chemotherapy.

The admission assessment reveals that Chris has a white blood count of 5100 and has had loose, greenish colored watery stools for the past two days. In the past six hours Chris has averaged three bowel movements per hour and complains "My tummy hurts." Chris had been eating well prior to this episode and has had no problem with nausea or vomiting according to his mother. The physician has concluded that the white blood count and liquid bowel movements are side effects from Chris' chemotherapy.

Your physical assessment finds a small reddened area over the sacral area as well as around the rectum and his bowel sounds are hyperactive. Chris states his "bottom is sore." Mrs. Appleton, during your interview states she has just urged Chris "to wipe himself good." Chris' mother says Chris has been remaining in bed due to feeling weak and dizzy and also reveals that Chris has been sleeping frequently during the day. Chris says, "I'm tired all the time." You note a pulse rate of 150 after you have helped Chris to the bathroom and back to bed. He also appears to have shortness of breath and a respiratory rate of 30.

Mrs. Appleton asks to speak with you privately. Chris states, "Mom's getting scared again so off she'll go." Mrs. Appleton tells Chris to shut up. During your interview with Mrs. Appleton she frequently asks for reassurance that Chris is going to get well. She says the doctor explained Chris' problem but she's just not going to believe it. She then talks about the problem not developing if she had taken Chris to the doctor sooner, if she had quit work sooner and stayed home with Chris rather than sending him to a day nursery to catch "bugs" or if she had made sure he ate a proper diet each day. She then tells you the real reason she wanted to talk to you is to inform the nursing staff she would be staying with Chris all the time and would be doing all his care since "We may lose him." She continues by saying, "Chris is too sick to help himself even though he tries; but, I don't want him getting too tired. One of these days I'll learn what to do for him."

HEALTH PERCEPTION-HEALTH MANAGEMENT PATTERN

Infection, Risk for (Page 43)

Risk Factors Present:

Inadequate primary defenses—change in pH of secretions, altered

peristalsis

Inadequate secondary defenses and immunosuppression—leukemia and

chemotherapy

Inadequate acquired immunity—inoculations delayed

Chronic disease—leukemia

Invasive procedures—I.V. chemotherapy

Pharmaceutical agents—Chemotherapy

Insufficient knowledge to avoid exposure—mother delayed bringing

to doctor for 2 days; inadequate care for rectal area "wipe

himself good".

NUTRITIONAL-METABOLIC PATTERN

Skin Integrity, Impaired: Risk for (Page 193)

Risk Factors Present:

Chemical substance—moisture, diarrhea

Mechanical factors—frequent sleeping (pressure, immobility)

Physical immobilization—self imposed due to "feeling tired"

Excretions—diarrheal stools

Medication—chemotherapy

Altered pigmentation—reddened area

Developmental factors--5 year old with chronic disease

Immunologic—leukemia plus chemotherapy plus delay in

inoculations

Altered circulation—chemotherapy I.V., immobilization, activity

intolerance

ELIMINATION PATTERN

Diarrhea (Page 223)

Defining Characteristics Present:

Abdominal pain/cramping—"My tummy hurts."

Increased frequency--three bowel movements per hour

Increased frequency of bowel sounds—auscultation revealed

hyperactive bowel sounds

Loose, liquid stools—admission information

Change in color—greenish colored

ACTIVITY-EXERCISE PATTERN

Activity Intolerance (Page 250)

Defining Characteristics Present:

Verbal report of fatigue or weakness—"I'm tired all the time."

Mother stated has been remaining in bed due to feeling weak and

dizzy.

Abnormal heart rate or blood pressure response to activity—

increased pulse rate

Exertional discomfort or dyspnea—increased respiratory rate,

shortness of breath

NOTE: STUDENTS MAY WISH TO USE DIAGNOSIS OF FATIGUE (PAGE 320);

HOWEVER, THE DEFINING CHARACTERISTICS FIT BEST WITH ACTIVITY

INTOLERANCE NOT FATIGUE.

SLEEP-REST PATTERN

No diagnoses related to this pattern.

COGNITIVE-PERCEPTUAL PATTERN

No diagnoses related to this pattern; however, students may want to

use Pain due to statement "My tummy hurts". This statement fits better with the diarrhea

diagnosis and would be subsumed under the therapies for the diarrhea.

Another diagnosis, under this pattern, students may want to use is

Knowledge Deficit for the Mother—"One of these days I'll know what

to do." While neither of these diagnoses would do any harm to the patient, combining the mother's statement with the other data she has

given indicates the Diagnosis of Family Coping, Ineffective: Compromised.

SELF-PERCEPTION AND SELF-CONCEPT PATTERN

No diagnoses related to this pattern. Students might want to use the

diagnosis Fear for the mother but, have the students combine all the data the

mother is giving and they will see the Diagnosis of Family Coping,

Ineffective: Compromised is more accurate.

ROLE-RELATIONSHIP PATTERN

No diagnosis related to this pattern. Students might want to use the

diagnosis Family Processes, Altered. Review of the defining characteristics for Altered

Family Processes will demonstrate Ineffective Family Coping:

Compromised is best.

SEXUALITY-REPRODUCTIVE PATTERN

No diagnoses related to this pattern.

COPING-STRESS TOLERANCE PATTERN

Family Coping, Ineffective: Compromised (Page 721)

Defining Characteristics Present:

Client expresses or confirms a concern or complaint about significant other's

response to his or her health problem—Chris' statement about "Mom's getting scared

again so off she'll go". Significant person describes preoccupation with personal reaction (e.g., fear, guilt, anticipatory grief, anxiety) to client's illness or disability or to other situational or development crises—entire last paragraph of case study.

Significant persons describes or confirms inadequate understanding or knowledge base which interferes with effective assistive or supportive behavior—last paragraph of case study.

Significant person displays protective behavior disproportionate (too little or too much) to the client's abilities or need for autonomy—will stay with all the time and would be doing all his care.

Family Coping, Ineffective: Disabled is not correct. The defining characteristics for this diagnosis are not present.

VALUE-BELIEF PATTERN

No diagnoses related to this pattern.

EXPECTED OUTCOMES AND TARGET DATES

Have students write own expected outcomes first then compare and contrast to the expected outcomes in the book. Risk for Infection, page 43; Impaired Skin Integrity: Risk for, page 193; Diarrhea, page 223 ; Activity Intolerance, page 250; and Ineffective Family Coping: Compromised, page 721.

NURSING ACTIONS

Refer students to appropriate pages in book. Have them select nursing actions pertinent for Chris and individualize these actions for Chris' age and condition.

EVALUATION

Use follow-up on next page. Again, have students group data according to each diagnosis. Refer the students to the appropriate evaluation decision flow sheet in the book. Have the students list the data collected as it relates to each expected outcome and then make decisions as to whether they are going to record REVISE, CONTINUE, or RESOLVED for each diagnosis.

The most appropriate decisions, based on the accompanying data, are:

Risk for Infection—may be either RESOLVED or CONTINUE. Chris is

not at risk now due to control of diarrhea, C.B.C. level in midrange and vital signs within normal range; therefore, students might make the decision the diagnosis has been resolved. CONTINUE could also be appropriate due to the medical diagnosis of leukemia and continuing chemotherapy.

Impaired Skin Integrity: Risk for—The most accurate decision

would be CONTINUE with a change in the target date as long as the reddened area still exists.

Diarrhea—RESOLVED. Chris has none of the defining characteristics

remaining for this diagnosis.

Activity Intolerance—RESOLVED. Chris has none of the defining

characteristics remaining for this diagnosis.

Ineffective Family Coping: Compromised—REVISE to Family Coping,

Potential for Growth (Page 730). Revise target date and nursing actions.

Add new nursing diagnosis of Anticipatory Grieving (Page 594).

FOLLOW-UP

CHRIS APPLETON

Chris has now been in the hospital 5 days. His white blood cell count has risen to 7,600. His temperature is 98.4 degrees F. orally, pulse 84, respiration 16 and regular and Blood pressure 128/86.

Chris is now having one bowel movement per day and it is of normal color and consistency. He continues to eat well and has no problems with nausea or vomiting. I and O measurement shows Chris' I and O to be within normal range.

Chris still has a reddened area over the sacral area; but, it has decreased in size. Chris no longer complains of his "bottom being sore." Chris is ambulating freely and has no shortness of breath or increase pulse rate after ambulating. He is now sleeping 10 hours at night with a 1 hour nap during the day.

Counseling with Chris' parents has resulted in their verbalization of a better understanding of the pathophysiology and prognosis of Chris' medical diagnosis. Mrs. Appleton still has a tendency to "hover" over Chris; but, both parents have been more assertive in their discussions with Chris' physician. The physician has indicated Chris will probably be discharged in 4-5 days. His parents are consulting with the nursing staff regarding plans for Chris' discharge. They are concerned over balancing Chris' activities, maintaining his comfort and safety in their home, preventing infections, obtaining necessary equipment and supplies at a reasonable cost, and maintaining good family relationships with Chris' older brother (age 11) and sister (age 8). They are going to attend the next meeting of the local Leukemia Support Group.

The physician has told Chris' parents that Chris is not responding well to the chemotherapy and there is little likelihood a remission is going to occur. Mr. and Mrs. Appleton can now talk about Chris' impending death although it is apparent it is still a very difficult, painful subject. Both can freely verbalize their distress when given an opportunity to do so but, still cannot verbalize well to each other. Both parents relate difficulty in concentrating on their activities of daily living, indicate they have difficulty sleeping and have to force themselves to eat. Mr. and Mrs. Appleton express varying levels of guilt, anger, and denial but, understand the reasons for their fluctuating emotions. Counselors working with Chris' siblings indicate his brother and sister are coping well with Chris' illness.

ANN BASTROW

Ann Bastrow is a 30-year-old woman who was admitted to the unit directly from the operating room. She was in a car accident this morning and was sent to surgery from the emergency room for a splenectomy and internal fixation of a compound fracture of the left leg. During surgery 1500 cc's of blood were suctioned from Ann's abdomen. She received two units of blood during surgery and has another unit infusing now. She has 5/DW with 15 mEq. of KCl infusing in the other arm. You see a note from the anesthesiologist urging caution when caring for Ann so that the I.V.s would not infiltrate. Her I.V. lines were very difficult to start due to decreased venous filling and venous filling has not significantly improved. Ann's hgb., hct. and Na are elevated.

It is now 1 a.m. Ann has a Foley catheter, which is draining 25 cc's of concentrated urine per hour. Ann's vital signs are: T. 103.6 degrees F. rectally, P. 100, R. 22 and B.P. 90/64. Her skin is flushed, very dry, and very warm to touch. Ann has decreased skin turgor and dry mucous membranes. Ann complains of being thirsty, feeling weak, and states her left side and leg hurt. She had Demerol 100 mg. I.M. 3 hours ago. She refuses to cough or deep breathe and is lying very still and rigid. Ann drifts in and out of sleep and complains that she cannot fall asleep. She is sleeping for no more than 30 minutes at a time. Ann says she cannot rest and is becoming increasingly irritable and lethargic. Her speech is slurred. She communicates in yes or no answers and occasionally answers inappropriately. She makes frequent facial grimaces. Her eyes appear dull, the pupils are dilated, and she has scattered eye movements. Ann refuses to use the overhead trapeze due to pain from the splenectomy incision and does not move unless someone turns her. She also complains of pain when passive range of motion exercises are attempted.

The physician left orders that Ann is to be on strict bed rest, may have clear liquids, may have Demerol 100 mg. I.M. every 3 hours p.r.n., is to have one more unit of whole blood, and the current I.V. in the other arm is to be followed by 1000 cc's of Ringer's Lactate solution to be given at a keep open rate.

NURSING DIAGNOSES ACCORDING TO PATTERNS

HEALTH PERCEPTION-HEALTH MANAGEMENT PATTERN

Ann has no nursing diagnoses in this pattern. Students may want to

use diagnoses of Altered Health Maintenance, Ineffective Management of

Therapeutic Regimen: Individual or Noncompliance but, the defining

characteristics for these diagnoses are not present.

NUTRITIONAL-METABOLIC PATTERN

Fluid Volume Deficit (Page 129)

Defining Characteristics Present:

Decreased urine output--25 cc's per hour

Concentrated urine

Decreased venous filling

Hemoconcentration—based on hgb. and hct. elevation

Increased serum sodium

Hypotension—B.P. of 90/64

Thirst—Patient statement

Increased pulse rate—P. of 100

Decreased skin turgor

Change in mental state—answers questions inappropriately, slurred

speech, irritability

Increased body temperature--103.6 degrees F. rectally

Dry skin

Dry mucous membrane

Weakness—patient statement

Hyperthermia (Page 145)

Defining Characteristics Present:

Increase in body temperature above normal range—Rectal

Temperature of 103.6 degree F.—Normal range for rectal

temperature range is generally considered to be 99.6 degrees plus

or minus one degree.

Flushed skin

Warm to touch

Increased respiratory rate—R. of 22

Tachycardia—P. of 100

ELIMINATION PATTERN

Ann has no diagnoses in this pattern. Students may want to use

Urinary Retention based on the decreased output; but, she does not

present the defining characteristics of Urinary Retention.

ACTIVITY-EXERCISE PATTERN

Impaired Physical Mobility, Level 3 (Page 362)

Defining Characteristics Present:

Inability to purposefully move within the physical environment,

including bed mobility, transfer, and ambulation—Refuses to use

trapeze, lying very still.

Reluctance to attempt movement—does not turn unless moved, refuses

to use trapeze, lying very still.

Limited range of motion—does not do, complains of pain when

passive range of motion exercises are attempted.

Imposed restrictions of movement, including mechanical, medical

protocol—strict bed rest, repair of compound fracture.

SLEEP-REST PATTERN

Sleep Pattern Disturbance (Page 397)

Defining Characteristics Present:

Verbal complaints of difficulty falling asleep—patient's statement.

Interrupted sleep—sleeping no more than 30 minutes at a time.

Verbal complaints of not feeling well rested—patient's statement.

Changes in behavior and performance—irritability, restlessness, lethargic

Thick speech with mispronunciation and incorrect words—slurred

speech, inappropriate answering of yes-no questions.

COGNITIVE-PERCEPTUAL PATTERN

<u>Pain, Acute</u> (Page 453)

Defining Characteristics Present:

Communication (verbal or coded) of pain descriptions—patient's statement.

Guarding behavior, protective—lying very still and rigid, refusal to move, won't use trapeze.

Narrowed focus—answers questions only yes or no, answers questions inappropriately.

Facial mask of pain—eyes dull, scattered movement of eyes, facial grimace.

Autonomic responses not seen in chronic stable pain—pupillary dilation, increased respiratory rate.

SELF-PERCEPTION AND SELF-CONCEPT PATTERN

No diagnoses in this pattern.

SEXUALITY-REPRODUCTIVE PATTERN

No diagnoses in this pattern.

COPING-STRESS TOLERANCE PATTERN

No diagnoses in this pattern.

VALUE-BELIEF PATTERN

No diagnoses in this pattern.

EXPECTED OUTCOMES AND TARGET DATES

Have students write own expected outcomes first, then compare and contrast to the expected outcomes in the book. Fluid Volume Deficit, page 129; Hyperthermia, page 145; Impaired Physical Mobility: Level 3, page 362; Sleep Pattern Disturbance, page 397 and Acute Pain, page 453.

NURSING ACTIONS

Refer students to appropriate pages in book. Have them select nursing actions appropriate for Ann and individualize these actions for her condition.

EVALUATION

Use follow-up on next page. Again, have students group data according to each diagnosis. Refer the students to the appropriate evaluation flow sheet in the book. Have the students list the data collected as it relates to each expected outcome and then make decisions as to whether they are going to record REVISE, CONTINUE, or RESOLVED for each diagnosis.

The most appropriate decisions based on the accompanying data are:

Fluid Volume Deficit—RESOLVED. Ann no longer has any defining characteristics for this diagnosis.

Hyperthermia—RESOLVED. Ann no longer has any defining characteristics for this diagnosis.

Impaired Physical Mobility: Level 3--REVISE to level 2 (requires help from another person). Change target date and nursing actions as necessary.

<u>Sleep</u> <u>Pattern</u> <u>Disturbance</u>—RESOLVED. Ann no longer has any defining

characteristics for this diagnosis.

<u>Acute Pain</u>—CONTINUE and change target date. Ann is still requiring some

pain medication.

Add Impaired Skin Integrity: Risk for (Page 193) and

Self Care, Deficit (Bathing-Hygiene, Dressing-Grooming) (Page 371).

FOLLOW-UP

ANN BASTROW

Ann was returned to surgery at 3:00 a.m. for control of continuing bleeding at the site of the splenectomy. She had no further bleeding problems. Ann has now been in the hospital for 7 days. Her hemoglobin is 12.8 and her vital signs are T. 98.6 degrees orally, P. 96, R 16 and B.P. 122/84. Her vital signs and hemoglobin level have remained stabilized for 4 days. Her I.V.s have been discontinued and she is maintaining a balanced intake and output.

The physician allows Ann to be up in a chair only twice a day for fifteen minutes each time. The last X-ray taken of her left leg demonstrated delayed healing of the fracture. Ann's complaints regarding pain have decreased and she only requires one analgesic about every 12-18 hours. She is now on an oral analgesic. Ann is sleeping from 10 p.m. to 7 a.m. without requiring a sleeping aid. She indicates no problems with sleeping.

Ann still requires a high degree of assistance in caring for herself. She can feed herself (general diet) and wash her upper body. The remainder of her needs have to be handled by the nurse. Ann does cooperate fully in turning, coughing, deep breathing, and in other activities to the degree she is capable.

In caring for Ann you note a small reddened area on her left posterior thigh just at the edge of the cast. The circulation and sensation, in the left leg, are normal.

Ann has begun to talk about going home and is asking you questions about maintaining her care at home. She has a housemate who will be there except from 8 a.m. to 5:30 p.m. due to her employment. The physician has indicated Ann will need to wear the cast for at least 6 more weeks and possibly longer. At this time the physician doubts Ann will be able to bear weight on the involved leg for at least 4 more weeks but could be discharged from the hospital prior to that time.

CASE STUDY 3

MR. FRED CARSON

Mr. Fred Carson is a 63-year-old man who has been admitted with a medical diagnosis of hyperglycemia secondary to diabetes mellitus. He was first diagnosed as having adult onset diabetes 2 years ago.

On admission, Mr. Carson's vital signs are: temperature 101.4 degrees F. orally, pulse 98, respiration 20, blood pressure 98/70. Mr. Carson is 5 feet 9 inches tall and weighs 230 pounds. He states he has gained 20 lbs. over the past 6 weeks. His fasting glucose is 200 mg/dL. His hgb. level is 20 g/dL. and an hct. of 56 vol/dL. Mr. Carson tells you he regulates his insulin according to what he eats and eats whatever he is hungry for. You find, in interviewing Mr. Carson, that he has been drinking 3 to 4 "ice tea glasses" of water every hour stating "I'm always thirsty." He has been voiding at least once an hour. His urine specimen is dilute and a very pale yellow. Mr. Carson's urine glucose, as measure by a clinitest, is 4+. In the past 2 hours Mr. Carson voided 1500 cc's in addition to the urine specimen and his intake has been 500 cc's. Mr. Carson says he doesn't pay any attention to his urine tests, "They're just a waste of time" but, does add "I've been peeing alot more that past few days. Does this mean I'm not behaving?" Mr. Carson states he was taught about his diabetes but thinks "They were just trying to scare me. I don't think I really have diabetes; kids develop that not old codgers like me. I only check in with the doc when I feel like it. He wants me to come in every other month but, I think he's just trying to get more money." When asked to discuss what he was taught regarding his diabetes Mr. Carson relates a high level of understanding of his prescribed regimen.

You find out this is Mr. Carson's fourth admission over the last 8 months. All of the admissions have been due to complications secondary to the diabetes. He exhibits anger on each admission and refused to have home health nurses visit him.

In examining Mr. Carson's skin you find that his toenails and finger nails are dry, thick, and brittle. Both his skin and mucous membranes are dry in spite of the amount of fluid Mr. Carson indicates he was drinking prior to admission. His extremities are shiny, cool to the touch, and his legs become cyanotic when they are kept in a dependent position. When elevated his legs become pale and color is very slow to return when his legs are returned to a neutral position. His pedal pulses are difficult to locate and diminished in volume. He has a 10 cm+ size lesion on his left shin and you can see that the lesion has begun to impact the muscle tissue. Mr. Carson tells you he hit his leg on a table 3 weeks ago. You note three round scars with atrophied skin on his right leg and one similar scar on his left leg. Mr. Carson describes a sensation of "pins and needles when walking but, if I stop it goes away."

NURSING DIAGNOSES ACCORDING TO PATTERNS

HEALTH PERCEPTION-HEALTH MANAGEMENT PATTERN

Noncompliance (Page 67)

Defining Characteristics Present:

Behaviors indicative of failure to adhere—self regulation of insulin, disregard of diet, weight, statements re urine testing, frequent admissions

Objective tests—blood glucose, urine tests

Evidence of development of complications—lab tests, extremities, leg lesion

Evidence of exacerbation of symptoms—lab tests, polydipsia, polyuria

Failure to keep appointments—statement regarding physician appointments

NUTRITIONAL-METABOLIC PATTERN

Fluid Volume Deficit (Page 129)

Defining Characteristics Present:

Dilute urine—observation of specimen

Increased urine output—output measurement for 2 hours, patient's statement

Weight gain—weighs 230 pounds, statement about weight gain

Hypotension—B.P. 98/70

Increased pulse rate—pulse rate of 98

Decreased pulse pressure--28 [98-70] versus 40 [120-80]

Increased body temperature--101.4 orally

Dry skin

Dry mucous membranes

Hemoconcentration—hgb. and hct. measurements

Thirst—patient's statements

Impaired Skin Integrity, Actual (Page 193)

Defining Characteristics Present:

Disruption of skin surface—lesion on left shin

Destruction of skin layers—lesion has begun invasion of muscle layer

ELIMINATION PATTERN

No diagnoses related to this pattern. Mr. Carson does have increased

urinary output but, does not have the defining characteristics for

incontinence.

ACTIVITY-EXERCISE PATTERN

Altered Tissue Perfusion (Page 380)

Defining Characteristics Present:

Extremities cool to touch—legs cool to touch

Extremities cyanotic when in dependent position—description of color changes in leg

Extremities pale on elevation, slow color return—description of color changes in leg

Diminished arterial pulsations—pedal pulses difficult to locate

Skin quality: Shining—description of legs' appearance

Round scars covered with atrophied skin—description of legs' appearance

Dry, thick, brittle nails—description of fingernails and toenails

Claudication—"pins and needles sensations" alleviated by rest

Slow healing of lesions—injury occurred 3 weeks ago—no evidence

of healing

SLEEP-REST PATTERN

No diagnoses related to this pattern

COGNITIVE-PERCEPTUAL PATTERN

No diagnoses related to this pattern

SELF-PERCEPTION AND SELF-CONCEPT PATTERN

No diagnoses related to this pattern

ROLE-RELATIONSHIP PATTERN

No diagnoses related to this pattern

SEXUALITY-REPRODUCTIVE PATTERN

No diagnoses related to this pattern

COPING-STRESS PATTERN

Impaired Adjustment (Page 704)

Defining Characteristics Present:

Verbalization of non acceptance of health status change—patient's statement regarding "I don't think I really have diabetes."

Unsuccessful ability to be involved in problem solving or goal setting—multiple admissions, noncompliance

Extended period of disbelief and anger—patient's statements

Lack of future oriented thinking—refuses home health care, noncompliance

VALUE-BELIEF PATTERN

No diagnoses related to this pattern

EXPECTED OUTCOMES AND TARGET DATE

Have students write own expected outcomes first then compare and contrast to the expected outcomes in the book. Noncompliance, page 67; Fluid Volume Deficit, page 129; Impaired Skin Integrity, page 193; Altered Tissue Perfusion, page 380 and Impaired Adjustment, page 704 .

NURSING ACTIONS

Refer students to appropriate pages in book. Have them select nursing actions pertinent for Mr. Carson and individualize those actions for Mr. Carson's age and condition.

EVALUATION

Use follow-up on next page. Again, have students group data according to each diagnosis. Refer the students to the appropriate evaluation decision flow sheet in the book. Have the students list the data collected as it relates to each expected outcome and then make decisions as to whether they are going to record REVISE, CONTINUE or RESOLVED for each diagnosis.

The most appropriate decisions, based on the accompanying data, are:

Noncompliance—RESOLVED, at this time. CONTINUE could also be appropriate due to Mr. Carson's statement regarding "lot of bother to keep up with all this stuff." This statement would indicate there is still the risk for noncompliance.

Fluid Volume Deficit—RESOLVED. Mr. Carson no longer demonstrates the defining characteristics for this diagnoses.

Impaired Skin Integrity, Actual—CONTINUE. The lesion on Mr. Carson's leg is improving but, it is still present. Change target date and nursing actions as necessary.

Altered Tissue Perfusion—RESOLVED. Mr. Carson no longer exhibits the defining characteristics for this diagnosis.

Impaired Adjustment—RESOLVED. Mr. Carson no longer presents the defining characteristics for this diagnosis.

Add Impaired Home Maintenance Management (Page 344)

128

FOLLOW-UP

MR. FRED CARSON

Mr. Carson has now been in the hospital for 6 days. His intake and output are balanced within normal limits and his vital signs have been stabilized within normal limits for the past 4 days. His blood and urine glucose levels are within normal limits.

Mr. Carson has lost 20 pounds, but complains about the diet although he is not doing any cheating on the diet. He can now correctly test his urine and administer his own insulin. Mr. Carson verbalizes his understanding about his insulin and urine tests and states he now "really knows why I kept getting into trouble. I didn't see the connections between all of these things." He still indicates however, that "it sure is a lot of bother to keep up with all of this stuff." He has signed a contract with you to keep his doctors' appointments, to test his urine, to follow the diabetic exchange diet and to take his insulin as ordered. He states, "You can rely on me. When I give my word like this, I keep it." He has agreed he needs the services of home health nurses and you have made this referral. The home health nurse has an appointment this afternoon with Mr. Carson for his home care assessment. The doctor plans to discharge Mr. Carson in 3 days.

Mr. Carson reveals that he lives in a one room efficiency apartment in a low income section of town. He states he doesn't worry about keeping the place clean. "I just empty trash and straighten up when I can't stand the sight and odor any more. It would be nice to have someone to help me with it." He laughs and says he's going to teach the cockroaches to carry out the trash. "They're big enough to!" Mr. Carson has a monthly income of $500 from social security. His rent is $250 and utilities average $120 per month.

With the weight loss and improved health status, Mr. Carson's skin lesion has decreased in size and is clean and dry with evidence of granulated tissue. His legs are warm and the pedal pulses are full and regular. He has no signs or symptoms of claudication. His legs maintain normal coloration regardless of position.

CASE STUDY 4

MRS. BETTY DAWMER

Mrs. Betty Dawmer is a 42-year-old woman who has been admitted via the E.R. with a medical diagnosis of urinary tract infection. She is a real estate agent and is particularly concerned because she has been experiencing involuntary passage of urine. She states she has always been able to delay urination until she had time to go to a restroom. "In my business, that is essential. I can't be running to the restroom every little bit while I'm showing buyers all over town." She states she has been voiding about once per hour and that she now has to hunt a bathroom as soon as she feels the need to void. "I don't always make it and that's very embarrassing." She is complaining of severe lower abdominal pain and a sensation of cramping. She has been having to get up 4 to 6 time per night to void and generally voids small amounts. Mrs. Dawmer is married but has no children.

After your initial admission assessment, you reenter Ms. Dawmer's room and find she is crying. She tells you her pain is terrible and it has been at least 6 hours since she had any medication for pain. She appears very listless and her face appears drawn into a permanent scowl. As you recheck her vital signs, she holds up her hands as though asking you not to touch her. You check her chart and find she was given Demerol 75mg. 3 hours ago in E.R.

Mrs. Dawmer has achieved pain relief and asks you if she can discuss a personal matter with you. When you reply yes, she asks if her physical problem could be what has been affecting her sexual life. She reports that she and her husband have had a very satisfactory sexual relationship but having been having problems for the past month.

Neither partner, according to Mrs. Dawmer, have been satisfied with their relationship and neither wants to try "any of that kinky stuff" in an attempt to achieve satisfaction. Mrs. Dawmer states this problem has begun to affect other aspects of their life.

Mrs. Dawmer says she hopes she will get extra rest in the hospital since she feels so tired. Upon further questioning, Mrs. Dawmer reports she usually slept 8 hours per night but, lately she has been having difficulty in going to sleep. "I guess I know I'm going to be up and down all night." She sleeps only 1 to 2 hours at a time and invariably awakes at 5:30 a.m. when she use to sleep until 7 a.m. You note dark circles under her eyes and a mild tremor of her hands.

Mrs. Dawmer reveals that this is the first time she has ever been hospitalized and that she is worried over what will happen to her. She asks numerous questions about everything that is done to or for her. She is restless, is perspiring and states she feels shaky. She speaks rapidly and keeps asking for reassurance that she will fully recover from this illness. Her temperature is 100.2 degree F. orally, pulse 86, respiration 20 and her B.P. is 130/80. Her skin is cool and pale and her pupils are dilated.

NURSING DIAGNOSIS ACCORDING TO PATTERNS

HEALTH PERCEPTION-HEALTH MANAGEMENT PATTERN

No diagnoses related to this pattern

NUTRITIONAL-METABOLIC PATTERN

No diagnoses related to this pattern

ELIMINATION PATTERN

Altered Urinary Elimination Pattern: Urge Incontinence (Page 229)

Defining Characteristics Present:

Urinary urgency—patient's statements

Frequency (voiding more often than every 2 hours)--patient's statement

Bladder contraction or spasm—patient's statements

Nocturia (more than 2 times per night)--patient's statement

Voiding in small amounts—patient's statement

ACTIVITY-EXERCISE PATTERN

No diagnoses related to this pattern

SLEEP-REST PATTERN

Sleep Pattern Disturbance (Page 397)

Defining Characteristics Present:

Verbal complaints of difficulty falling asleep—patient's statement

Awakening earlier or later than desired—patient's statement

Interrupted sleep—patient's statement

Verbal complaints of not feeling well rested—patient's statement

Physical signs—dark circles under eye, hand tremor

COGNITIVE-PERCEPTUAL PATTERN

Acute Pain (Page 453)

Defining Characteristics Present:

Communication (verbal or coded) of pain descriptions—patient's statement

Guarding behavior, protective—hand gestures

Narrowed focus—altered time perception--6 hours since had pain mediation

Distraction behavior—crying

Facial mask of pain—facial scowl

Autonomic responses not seen in chronic stable pain—perspiration, blood pressure and

pulse measurements, pupillary dilation, increased respiration rate

SELF-PERCEPTION AND SELF-CONCEPT PATTERN

Anxiety (Page 496)

There are twenty-nine defining characteristics for this diagnosis.

Rather than take up space listing all the ones Mrs. Dawmer exhibits,

we assure you she demonstrates enough of the characteristics to lead

Students to this diagnosis. See page 497 to assist students in

differentiating between anxiety and fear.

ROLE-RELATIONSHIP PATTERN

No diagnoses related to this pattern

SEXUALITY-REPRODUCTIVE PATTERN

Sexual Dysfunction (Page 684)

Defining Characteristics Present:

Verbalization of problem—patient's statement

Actual or perceived limitation imposed by disease or therapy—patient's question regarding role of illness in problem

Conflicts involving values—statement regarding "kinky things"

Alteration in achieving sexual satisfaction—patient's statements

Inability to achieve desired satisfaction—patient's statements

Alteration in relationship with significant other—patient's statements

COPING-STRESS TOLERANCE PATTERN

No diagnoses related to this pattern

VALUE-BELIEF PATTERN

No diagnoses related to this pattern

EXPECTED OUTCOMES AND TARGET DATE

Have students write own expected first then compare and contrast to the expected outcomes in the book. Altered Urinary Elimination Pattern: Urge Incontinence, page 229

; Sleep Pattern Disturbance, page 397 ; Acute Pain, page   453 ; Anxiety, page 496 and Sexual Dysfunction, page 684.

NURSING ACTIONS

Refer students to appropriate pages in book. Have them select nursing actions pertinent for Mrs. Dawmer and individualize those actions for Mrs. Dawmer's situation.

EVALUATION

Use follow-up on next page. Again, have students group data according to each diagnosis. Refer the students to the appropriate evaluation decision flow sheet in the book. Have the students list the data collected as it relates to each expected outcome and then make decisions as to whether they are going to record REVISE, CONTINUE, or RESOLVED for each diagnosis.

The most appropriate decisions, based on the accompanying data, are:

Altered Urinary Elimination Pattern: Urge Incontinence—RESOLVED. Mrs. Dawmer no longer has any defining characteristics for this diagnosis.

Sleep Pattern Disturbance—RESOLVED. Mrs. Dawmer presents no defining characteristics for this diagnosis.

Acute Pain—RESOLVED. Mrs. Dawmer no longer exhibits any defining characteristics in this area.

Anxiety—CONTINUE. Mrs. Dawmer continues to exhibit some anxiety through her questioning and other statements. Change target date and nursing actions as necessary.

Sexual Dysfunction—CONTINUE. The Dawmer's are demonstrating progress toward

resolution of this problem; but, it is not resolved as yet.

With Mrs. Dawmer being scheduled for discharge tomorrow, there is

probably very little intervention you can do, but encourage continuation of the counseling.

Add Diversional Activity Deficit (Page 301)

FOLLOW-UP

MRS. BETTY DAWMER

Mrs. Dawmer has been in the hospital for 5 days. Her urinalyses demonstrates no signs of infection and her vital signs have remained within normal limits for 3 days. Mrs. Dawmer has had no complaints of pain for 48 hours and is sleeping continuously from 11 p.m. to 7 a.m. without the use of sleep medication.

She has had no episodes of incontinence since the infection began to clear. Her intake and output are balanced and she no longer has nocturia.

She states she is getting bored. She doesn't like watching television "those soap operas drive me nuts." She has no hobbies as such but considers bowling and tennis playing as her hobbies. She still frequently questions any activities related to her care but states she "not quite as scared as I was." She asks about the possible recurrence of her problem and has had you make a written list of all she could do to prevent a recurrence. She has had you go through the list three times with her to be sure she understands the regimen.

Mrs. Dawmer and her husband have had one counseling session, while she was in the hospital, regarding their sexual problems. The physician has explained that her UTI could have contributed to the problem. The couple indicate they will continue counseling until they feel comfortable the problem has been settled. Mrs. Dawmer is scheduled to be released from the hospital in 2 to 3 days.

CASE STUDY 5

JESSICA KEYMEYER

Jessica Keymeyer is a 16-year-old woman who is being admitted with a medical diagnosis of possible anorexia nervosa. Jessica's mother reports that Jessica became concerned about her weight 3 months ago. Since that time she eats only ½ cup of cottage cheese three times a day. Jessica is 5 feet 7 inches tall and weighs 92 pounds. She has lost 40 pounds in the last three months. Jessica's mother states if they make Jessica eat, Jessica then goes to the bathroom and makes herself vomit. Mrs. Keymeyer reports that Jessica now has a problem swallowing. Jessica states "Nothing tastes good" and "The cottage cheese fills me up." After further questioning, Jessica tells you she has episodes of abdominal cramping and pain. Jessica repeats several times that she is too fat. She refuses to look at herself in the mirror. She say fat girls don't get invited anyplace. "When I was in elementary, I had lots of friends. In Junior High I gained weight and no body wanted a fatso around." Jessica refuses to touch her arms or legs when you try to demonstrate the decreased muscle tone and mass. Her mother states Jessica only wears nonfitted clothes because "that's what fat girls wear." Jessica's mother also reports Jessica has cut off contact with her school friends "until I am fit to be seen with them."

As you interview Jessica you find out Jessica has not voided for 24 hours except for "a few dribbles." She states she feels like she needs to but "just can't" and is "too weak to walk to the bathroom." Her bladder appears distended and when you palpate the bladder area Jessica complains of pain.

Jessica appears emaciated and tells you she has spent most of the last 5 days in bed. Jessica is very reluctant to turn and to perform active range of motion. As you perform passive range of motion you find limitation in extension of the elbows and knees.

When she tries to ambulate, she is uncoordinated and you can readily see decreased muscle

mass. In examining Jessica you find an open, abraded area on the left buttock. Her

conjunctiva and mucous membranes are pale with two patches of ulceration in the left

buccal area. She has another lesion just inside the left nostril and one at the upper right

corner of her lips. Jessica has poor muscle tone and complains of hair loss. She has

decreased skin turgor and her skin and mucous membranes are dry. Jessica's vital signs

are temperature 101.8 degrees F. orally, pulse 84, respiration 20 and B.P. 92/80.

NURSING DIAGNOSES ACCORDING TO PATTERNS

HEALTH PERCEPTION-HEALTH MANAGEMENT PATTERN

No diagnoses in this pattern

NUTRITIONAL-METABOLIC PATTERN

Altered Nutrition: Less than Body Requirements (Page 163)

Defining Characteristics Present:

Body weight 20% or more under ideal--92 pounds, 5'7" tall, ideal weight would be closer to 130 pounds

Reported inadequate food intake less than RDA--1/2 cup cottage cheese three times per day

Weakness of muscles required for swallowing or mastication—mother's statement regarding Jessica's problem with swallowing

Reported or evidence of lack of food—see above

Satiety immediately after ingesting food—"fills me up"

Aversion to eating—several patient statements related to

Abdominal pain with or without pathology—Jessica's statement re cramping and pain

Sore, inflamed buccal cavity—presence of lesions

Abdominal cramping—Jessica's statement

Lack of interest in food—Jessica's statements

Pale conjunctival and mucous membranes—assessment findings

Poor muscle tone—assessment findings, difficulty in ambulation

Excessive loss of hair—Jessica's statement

Impaired Tissue Integrity (Page 193)

Defining Characteristics Present:

Damaged or destroyed tissue (cornea, mucous membrane,

integumentary, or subcutaneous)--abraded area on left buttock, lesions in

mouth, lesion on lip, lesion inside left nostril

ELIMINATION PATTERN

Urinary Retention (Page 237)

Defining Characteristics Present:

Bladder distention—assessment finding

Absence of urine output—has not voided for past 24 hours

Sensation of bladder fullness—Jessica's statement

Dribbling—Jessica's statement

Dysuria—Jessica's statement

ACTIVITY-EXERCISE PATTERN

Impaired Physical Mobility: Level 2 (Page 362)

Defining Characteristics Present:

Inability to purposefully move within the physical environment, including bed mobility, transfer and ambulation—has spent most of last 5 days in bed, incoordination, reluctant to move

Reluctance to attempt movement—too weak to go to bathroom, reluctant to turn in bed, reluctance to perform active ROM

Limited range of motion—limitation found in extension of knees and elbows

Decreased muscle strength, contact and mass—assessment findings of

decreased muscle mass, spent most of time in bed, too weak to go

to bathroom

Impaired coordination—observation when assisted Jessica to bathroom

SLEEP-REST PATTERN

No diagnoses in this pattern

COGNITIVE-PERCEPTUAL PATTERN

No diagnoses in this pattern

SELF-PERCEPTION AND SELF-CONCEPT PATTERN

Body Image Disturbance (Page 506)

Defining Characteristics Present:

Actual change in structure or function—loss of 40 pounds, emaciated appearance, below ideal weight, loss of muscle mass

Not looking at body part (intentional or unintentional)--refuses to look at self in mirror

Change in social involvement—has cut off contact with school friends

Not touching body part—refused to touch arms and legs

Hiding or overexposing body part (intentional or unintentional)--wears nonfitted clothes

Change in life-style—mother's and Jessica's statements

Fear or rejection or of reaction by others—multiple statements by Jessica

Negative feelings about body—multiple statements by Jessica

Refusal to verify actual change—multiple statements by Jessica indicating she still sees herself as fat

ROLE-RELATIONSHIP PATTERN

No diagnoses in this pattern

SEXUALITY-REPRODUCTIVE PATTERN

No diagnoses in this pattern

COPING-STRESS TOLERANCE PATTERN

No diagnoses in this pattern. Students may be inclined to use the

diagnosis Ineffective Individual Coping for Jessica but the defining

characteristics presented by Jessica are more descriptive of

Body Image Disturbance.

VALUE-BELIEF PATTERN

No diagnoses in this pattern

EXPECTED OUTCOMES AND TARGET DATE

Have students write own expected outcomes first then compare and contrast to the expected outcomes in the book. Altered Nutrition: Less than Body Requirements, page 163; Impaired Tissue Integrity, page 193; Urinary Retention, page 237; Impaired Physical Mobility, Level 2, page 362 and Body Image Disturbance, page 506.

NURSING ACTIONS

Refer students to appropriate pages in book. Have them select nursing actions pertinent for Jessica and individualize those actions for Jessica according to her developmental level and condition.

EVALUATION

Use follow-up on next page. Again, have students group data according to each diagnosis. Refer the students to the appropriate evaluation decision flow sheet in the book. Have the students list the data collected as it relates to each expected outcome and then make decisions as to whether they are going to record REVISE, CONTINUE, or RESOLVED for each diagnosis.

The most appropriate decisions, based on the accompanying data, are:

Altered Nutrition: Less than Body Requirements—CONTINUE. Jessica has sufficient fluid intake, but is eating only ½ of her diet, has to be observed closely or will make self vomit, is not within normal body weight range. Change target date and nursing actions as necessary.

Impaired Tissue Integrity—REVISE to Impaired Skin Integrity. The nasal, buccal and lip lesions have healed. The buttock abrasion has improved but is still present. Change target date and nursing actions as necessary.

<u>Urinary</u> <u>Retention</u>—RESOLVED. Jessica no longer presents any of the defining characteristics for this diagnosis.

<u>Impaired</u> <u>Physical</u> <u>Mobility</u>—RESOLVED. Jessica no longer presents any of the defining characteristics for this diagnosis.

<u>Body</u> <u>Image</u> <u>Disturbance</u>—CONTINUE. Jessica is still making multiple statements regarding her weight. Her reluctance to make eye contact, body posture, and self production of vomiting indicates this diagnosis is still very active. Change target date and nursing actions as necessary.

FOLLOW-UP

JESSICA KEYMEYER

Jessica has now been in the hospital for 10 days and has been transferred to the adolescent mental health unit. She is now taking fluids (water, diet coke and skimmed milk) in sufficient volume, is voiding normally, and her intake and output have been within normal limits for the past 4 days. Her vital signs are within normal limits. Jessica now weight 99 pounds. Jessica is ambulating frequently and no longer feels weak. She can demonstrate total ROM with no problems. Collaboration between the Psychiatric Nurse Practitioner, Physical Therapist and Diet Therapist has resulted in Jessica exercising at a normal level.

Jessica still expresses concern over getting "too fat" but verbalizes understanding of a basic, balanced diet. She plans her diet each day but only eats approximately ½ of each serving. She has to be observed closely or she will slip off to the bathroom and make herself vomit.

In counseling sessions, Jessica refuses to make eye contact, sits hunched over and makes frequent statements related to "nobody really likes a fat person; it doesn't make any difference what you're really like." "Fat people are always slobs." "I like to eat but I can't afford to." "My old boyfriend liked skinny girls and dropped me when I got fat." "I go on eating binges when I get upset or feel sad and then I have to make myself vomit."

The lesion on Jessica's left buttock has decreased in size, is less inflamed appearing and granulating tissue has begun to form. Her conjunctiva and mucous membranes are normal in color and all of the lesions in the mouth, nostril and on the lip have healed. Her skin turgor is normal and her hair loss has stopped.

147

CASE STUDY 6

MRS. EMMA WATSON

Mrs. Emma Watson is a 67-year-old retired school teacher. She is a widow and lives by herself in a very nice three bedroom home. Her only child lives in England, but her younger sister lives next door to her. Mrs. Watson was admitted to the coronary care unit with a medical diagnosis of congestive heart failure.

The admission assessment shows that Mrs. Watson has pitting edema of her ankles (+4) and in the sacral area of her back (+2). As you auscultate her chest you hear moist rales and multiple rhonchi. Mrs. Watson coughs frequently with the production of a frothy sputum. You note that her jugular veins are very distended. Her peripheral pulses are difficult to locate and there is a 12 beat difference between the peripheral pulse rate and the apical rate (Apical = 84; peripheral = 72). Her other vital signs are T. 98 degrees F. orally, R. = 24 and B.P. 180/110. Mrs. Watson's skin is cool and clammy to the touch. Mrs. Watson is obviously short of breath and tells you breathes better when she is sitting upright. She sleeps on four pillows each night. She states she sleeps fairly well but lately she has been having dreams about dying that wake up her "scared nearly to death." She also has dreams about various disasters and some "are so weird they don't even make sense." Her monitor tracings show frequent PVCs and intermittent episodes of atrial fibrillation.

Mrs. Watson says she makes sure she drinks at least eight glasses of water per day—"that's what I always taught my students". She estimates these are 8 oz. glasses. In addition, she drinks at least two mugs of coffee with breakfast (approx. 8 oz. each), a small glass of orange juice with breakfast (approx. 4 oz. glass) plus iced tea at lunch and dinner (8 oz. glass). For the past 3 days she has been voiding no more than 3 times per day—"about a pint each time." When Mrs. Watson voided for her urine specimen, there was only 100 cc's of urine. She has voided 200 cc's. since that time. Palpation of the bladder does not demonstrate any bladder distention. She reports she has gained 10 pounds over the past 10 days and asks you if this could be fluid.

Mrs. Watson's chest x-ray show congestion in both lower lobes. Her lab tests show the following results: hgb.-8 g/dL, hct. 30%, Na-160 mEq/L, Ca-5.0 mEq/L, Cl-120 mEq/L, and K-6.0 mEq/L.

Mrs. Watson is constantly moving her legs and turns frequently from side to side. She states "I feel so tired but I just can't get comfortable." She complains of weakness and dizziness when she tries to ambulate to the bathroom. Her sister reports that Mrs. Watson has fainted twice in the past two days. You take Mrs. Watson's blood pressure after she returned from the bathroom and it was 110/84. After she has rested for awhile, a repeat blood pressure measurement shows it to be 170/100.

You notice as you interview Mrs. Watson that she frequently answers "Huh?" or responds incorrectly. She asks you why you are mumbling. She answers you with very short, sharp replies and you note she frequently clenches her hands while you are gathering data. Mrs. Watson's sister tells you Mrs. Watson can't hear well but refuses to admit it. "Emma gets so mad at me when I try to talk to her and asks me if I have mush in my mouth." The sister reports that Mrs. Watson refuses to go out and doesn't want friends to come over. "She used to belong to several clubs and entertained frequently but says it's too much trouble now." Mrs. Watson speaks in a monotone with a flat affect. She usually talks only when she is asked a direct question but tells you she will do anything you tell me to do. You note she generally closes her eyes when someone enters the room. Mrs. Watson tells you she doesn't go out much because "it's too crowded and people are rude. Besides my sister can get me whatever I need or I can have it delivered." She expresses sadness over her current state. "Nobody really wants me and I don't need anyone. You'll find out when you get old that society really doesn't have any use for you. Since I've retired I'm not much use to anybody." She says she doesn't understand why all of this illness is happening to her. "I've tried to be a good Christian person and look how I've wound up. I guess God doesn't really care for me after all. Surely a caring God wouldn't let one of his chosen to go through things like this." You soon learn that she has been physically unable to attend church for several months. You give her information about the chaplaincy services available and she asks you to have the Methodist minister to visit her.

NURSING DIAGNOSIS ACCORDING TO PATTERNS

HEALTH PERCEPTION-HEALTH MANAGEMENT PATTERN

No diagnoses related to this pattern.

NUTRITIONAL-METABOLIC PATTERN

Fluid Volume Excess (Page 137)

Defining Characteristics Present:

Edema—pitting edema of ankles and back, moist rales in lung, lung congestion

Effusion—moist rales in lungs

Anasarca—same data as listed for edema

Weight gain--10 pounds gained over past 10 days

Shortness of breath—Patient statement and observation

Orthopnea—Patient statement; sleeping on 4 pillows

Intake greater than output—Patient's daily intake versus voiding no more than 3 times per day (about a pint each time)

Pulmonary congestion—Chest x-ray

Abnormal breath sound—rales, rhonchi

Rales (crackles)--assessment results

Decreased hemoglobin and hematocrit—lab results

Blood pressure changes—B.P. 180/110; drops after ambulation; returns to high level after rest.

Jugular vein distention—observation

Oliguria—Last two voidings less than 100 cc's.

Altered electrolytes—Lab results

Restlessness—Observation

Anxiety—patient's statements

ELIMINATION PATTERN

No diagnoses in this pattern

ACTIVITY-EXERCISE PATTERN

Decreased Cardiac Output (Page 277)

Defining Characteristics Present:

Variations in blood pressure readings—variation before and after ambulation with rise after resting

Arrhythmias—PVCs, intermittent atrial fibrillation

Fatigue—patient's statement

Jugular vein distention—observation

Oliguria—last two voidings 100 cc's or below

Decreased peripheral pulses—pedal pulse assessments

Cold, clammy skin—assessment

Rales—chest assessment

Dyspnea, orthopnea—signs and symptoms of orthopnea

Restlessness—observation, patient's statements

Shortness of breath—patient's statement and observation

Syncope—Sister's report of patient's fainting

Vertigo—Patient's complaints of dizziness

Edema—pitting edema, pleural effusion, lung congestion

Cough—observation

Frothy sputum—observation

Weakness—patient's statement

SLEEP-REST PATTERN

No diagnoses in this pattern

COGNITIVE-PERCEPTUAL PATTERN

Sensory-Perceptual Alteration: Auditory (Page 465)

Defining Characteristics Present:

Reported or measured change in sensory acuity—Sister's statement, observation

Changes in behavior pattern—doesn't go out; doesn't entertain

Anxiety—patient's statements

Apathy—flat affect, will do what you tell her to; posture

Change in usual response to stimuli—replies to questions, limited socialization

Restlessness—observation

Irritability—anger toward sister; short, sharp answers, clenching of hands

Altered communication patterns—decreased socialization, way replies to question—remember, she was a school teacher

Complaints of fatigue—patient's statement

Inappropriate responses—"Huh?"; incorrect answers

SELF-PERCEPTION AND SELF-CONCEPT PATTERN

No diagnoses in this pattern

ROLE-RELATIONSHIP PATTERN

Social Isolation (Page 645)

Defining Characteristics Present:

Has sad, dull affect—patient's statements, replies to questions

Is uncommunicative, withdrawn, no eye contact—closes eyes, replies to questions, decreased socialization

Projects hostility in voice and behavior—demonstrates anger

Seeks to be alone or exists in a subculture—does not go out; does not entertain

Has evidence of physical or mental handicap or altered state of wellness-hearing loss, congestive heart failure, other nursing diagnoses

Expresses feelings of aloneness imposed by others—patient's statements

Expresses feelings of rejection—patient's statements

Feels inadequacy in or absence of significant purpose in life—patient's statements

Feels insecurity in public—patient's statements

SEXUALITY-REPRODUCTIVE PATTERN

No diagnoses in this pattern

COPING-STRESS TOLERANCE PATTERN

No diagnoses in this pattern

VALUE-BELIEF PATTERN

Spiritual Distress (Distress of Human Spirit) (Page 757)

Defining Characteristics Present:

Expresses anger toward God—patient's statements

Questions meaning of suffering—patient's statements

Verbalizes concern about relationship with deity—patient's statements

Questions meaning of own existence—patient's statements

Is unable to participate in usual religious practices—has been unable to attend church

Seeks spiritual assistance—ask you to notify Methodist minister

Describes nightmares or sleep disturbances—patient's statements

Has alteration in behavior or mood evidenced by anger, crying, withdrawal, preoccupation, anxiety, hostility, apathy, and so forth.—patients statements and observed behavior

EXPECTED OUTCOMES AND TARGET DATE

Have students write own expected outcomes first then compare and contrast to the expected outcomes in the book. Fluid Volume Excess, page 137; Decreased Cardiac

155

Output, page 277; Sensory-Perceptual Alteration: Auditory, page 465; Social Isolation, page 645 and Spiritual Distress (Distress of Human Spirit), page 757.

NURSING ACTIONS

Refer students to appropriate pages in book. Have them select nursing actions pertinent for Mrs. Watson and individualize those actions for Mrs. Watson according to her developmental level and condition.

EVALUATION

Use follow-up on next page. Again, have students group data according to each diagnosis. Refer the students to the appropriate evaluation decision flow sheet in the book. Have the students list the data collected as it relates to each expected outcome and then make decisions as to whether they are going to record REVISE, CONTINUE, or RESOLVED for each diagnosis.

The most appropriate decisions, based on the accompanying data, are:

Fluid Volume Excess—RESOLVED. Mrs. Watson no longer has any of the defining characteristics for this diagnosis.

Decreased Cardiac Output—CONTINUE. Mrs. Watson has enlarged ventricles. Doctor's statements indicate this will be a permanent problem for Mrs. Watson.

Sensory-Perceptual Alteration: Auditory—RESOLVED. Fitting with hearing aid and pleased with results.

Social Isolation—RESOLVED. Patient's statements about getting out and about, surprising friends, and so forth.

<u>Spiritual</u> <u>Distress</u> (Distress of Human Spirit)--RESOLVED. Patient's statements, plans to attend church.

FOLLOW-UP

MRS. EMMA WATSON

Mrs. Watson has been in the hospital for 12 days and has been moved to a general adult health unit. Her vital signs are all remaining stable and have been stable for 4 days. X-rays and lab tests are all within normal range and her ECGs no longer show any atrial fibrillation or PVCs. The physician states her ventricles are enlarged and she will continue to have problems but adds the problems should be minor as long as she follows her prescribed diet, medication, and exercise regimen. Her intake and output are balanced and she no longer exhibits edema. Her lungs are clear when auscultated.

Through the efforts of her pastor and her sister, Mrs. Watson agreed to be fitted for a hearing aid. She is astonished at the results and calls herself an "old fool" for not seeking help before. She jokes about vanity and expresses definite plans to "be out and about as soon as I can. Boy, are some of my friends going to be shocked. They'll accuse me of being a swinger." She also expresses comfort with "my God. I guess I panicked when I was so ill. You know I really have been blessed. My sister is going with me to church each Sunday as soon as the doctor says it's o.k."

CASE STUDY 7

JOSEPH WILSON

Mr. Joseph Wilson, age 35, was admitted to the intensive care unit five days ago following surgery for a depressed skull fracture and evacuation of a subdural hematoma. Mr. Wilson was in an automobile accident in which his car was hit from the rear by a drunken driver. Mr. Wilson was not wearing his seat belt at the time of the accident and his head impacted with the windshield. Mr. Wilson's wife, who was in the car with him and who was wearing her seat belt escaped the accident with a few minor lacerations and abrasions.

Mr. Wilson's current vital signs are T.-99.4 degrees F. tympanically, P.- 84 radial, regular, R.-18 diaphragmatic, on a ventilator, B.P. 134/88, left arm, lying down. Mr. Wilson has begun to assist with respirations. Over the last four days, Mr. Wilson's temperature has fluctuated between 96.4 degrees F. and 101.6 degrees F. During these temperature shifts, his skin has been alternatively cool and pale with slow capillary refill and cyanotic nails beds to warm to touch and flushing. His heart rate and respirations have also increased during these episodes. There have been no seizures or convulsions. Mr. Wilson is on phenytoin as a precaution against seizures.

Mr. Wilson weighs 185 pounds and is 6'0" tall. Mrs. Wilson reports that Mr. Wilson has no allergies to medicine or food.

Mr. Wilson is currently restless and irritable but is fairly cooperative when given direct instructions. Mrs. Wilson is anxious about her husband's condition and expresses anger that God would let this happen to her husband. She also wonders why she was spared and her husband was so mutilated.

Mr. Wilson exhibits loss of deep tendon reflexes on the right side (his dominant side), does not respond to sensation (sharp, dull, hot, cold, or light touch). He positions himself in bed using his left arm and leg but is unable to safely position his right arm and leg. Mr. Wilson is unwilling to do any self care for the right side. Small fasciculations are noted in the right arm and leg and he is unable to voluntarily move muscles of the right arm or leg. He shows only slight resistance to pressure.

CRANIAL NERVE CHECKS

1.   intact

2.   intact

3.   Lt intact; Rt-ptosis of eyelid; pupils equal, round, and reactive to

      light and accommodation.

4.   Lt intact; Rt-remains at midline.

5.   Lt intact; Rt-diminished muscle tone of temporal and masseter

      muscles; absence of sensation; does blink when cornea is touched.

6.   Lt intact; Rt-remains at midline.

7.   Lt intact; Rt-mouth pulls away from right side when asked to smile;

      Rt cheek puffs out on expiration.

8.   intact

9.   intact

10.   intact

11. Lt intact; Rt-unable to shrug shoulder or turn head against

resistance.

12. intact

Mr. Wilson is receiving 1500 mL of D_5NS a day and is receiving tube feedings

every four hours. His bowel sounds are sluggish. Mrs. Wilson reports that Mr. Wilson

generally has a bowel movement every day. Mr. Wilson indicates, via a magic slate, that

he feels bloated, has pressure in his rectum, and feels like he has to have a bowel

movement. Dulcolax tab 1, via the feeding tube, has been given for the last two nights

without results. A hard formed stool is palpable on digital exam.

The nurse is attempting to wean Mr. Wilson from the ventilator. Mr. Wilson

becomes pale, restless and diaphoretic. He indicates that he is apprehensive, expresses

that he is not getting enough oxygen and has a "wide-eyed" look. He watches the nurse's

every movement. Mr. Wilson is increasingly concentrating on every breath. Breathing has

changed from diaphragmatic to abdominal with slight use of accessory muscles. His vital

signs have increase to P-108, R-28, and BP 152/98. Mr. Wilson does not respond well to

coaching.

Mrs. Wilson has spent the majority of time at the hospital since her husband's

surgery. She wonders if Mr. Wilson will every regain use of his right side. She states that

he is a carpenter and that he will not be able to work if he does not fully recover. Both she

and Mr. Wilson attend church regularly and pray together; but, she is questioning why her

prayers have not been answered and why her husband has to suffer so much. She has been

to see her minister and the hospital chaplain has visited her; however, she expresses anger with them. She states, "They are God's chosen ones. Why doesn't God help my husband."

NURSING DIAGNOSES ACCORDING TO PATTERNS

HEALTH PERCEPTION-HEALTH MANAGEMENT PATTERN

No diagnoses in this pattern

NUTRITIONAL-METABOLIC PATTERN

Thermoregulation, Ineffective (page 188)

Defining Characteristics Present

Fluctuations in body temperature above or below the normal range

Hyperthermia (page 145)

Defining Characteristics Present

Increased temperature above normal

Flushed skin

Warm to touch

Increased respiratory rate

Increased heart rate

Hypothermia (page 152)

Defining Characteristics Present

Decreased temperature below normal

Shivering

Cool skin

Pallor

Slow capillary refill

Tachycardia

Cyanotic nail beds

ELIMINATION PATTERN

Constipation (page 216)

Defining Characteristics Present

Decreased activity level

Frequency less than usual pattern

Hard formed stool

Reported feeling of pressure in rectum

Reported feeling of rectal fullness

Abdominal pain

Appetite impairment

Use of laxatives

ACTIVITY-EXERCISE PATTERN

Dysfunctional Ventilatory Weaning Response (Page 308)

Defining Characteristics Present

Restlessness

Increase in BP, P and R from baseline

Expressed feelings of increased need for oxygen

Breathing discomfort

Increased concentration of breathing

Hypervigilence to activities

Inability to respond to coaching

Apprehension

Diaphoresis

Wide-eyed look

Slight use of respiratory accessory muscles

SLEEP-REST PATTERN

No diagnoses related to this pattern

COGNITIVE-PERCEPTUAL PATTERN

Unilateral Neglect (page 485)

Defining Characteristics Present

Consistent inattention to stimuli on an affected side

Inadequate self-care

Positioning and/or safety precautions in regard to affected side

SELF-PERCEPTION AND SELF-CONCEPT PATTERN

No diagnoses related to this pattern. Students may want to use

several of the diagnoses in this pattern; however, there is not

enough data given to support any of the diagnoses in this pattern.

ROLE-RELATIONSHIP PATTERN

No diagnoses related to this pattern. Students may want to use the

diagnoses of Altered Family Processes, Dysfunctional Grieving, or

Altered Role Performance. There is not enough data given to support

these diagnoses.

SEXUALITY-REPRODUCTIVE PATTERN

No diagnoses related to this pattern.

COPING-STRESS TOLERANCE PATTERN

No diagnoses related to this pattern. Students may want to use the

diagnosis of Ineffective Individual Coping; however, the defining

characteristics better fit with Spiritual Distress.

VALUE BELIEF PATTERN

Spiritual Distress (page 757)

Defining Characteristics Present

Expresses concern with meaning of life/death and/or belief systems

Anger toward God

Questions meaning of suffering

Verbalized inner conflicts about beliefs

Verbalized concern about relationship with deity

Questions meaning of own existence

Seeks spiritual assistance

Displacement of anger toward religious representatives

Alteration in behavior/mood evidenced by anger, crying, withdrawal,

Preoccupation, anxiety, hostility, apathy, etc.

EXPECTED OUTCOMES AND TARGET DATES

Have students write own expected outcomes first then compare and contrast to the
expected outcomes in the book. Ineffective Thermoregulation, page 188; Constipation,
page 216 ; Unilateral Neglect, page 485 ; Dysfunctional Ventilatory Weaning Response,
page 308 ; Spiritual Distress, page 757 .

NURSING ACTIONS

Refer students to appropriate pages in books. Have them select nursing actions
appropriate for Mr. and Mrs. Wilson and individualize these actions for Mr. Wilson's
condition.

EVALUATION

Use the follow-up on the next page. Again, have students group data according to
each diagnosis. Refer the students to the appropriate evaluation decision flow sheet in the
book. Have the students list the collected data as it relates to each expected outcome and
then make decisions as to whether they are going to record REVISE, CONTINUE, or
RESOLVED for each diagnosis.

The most appropriate decisions, based on the accompanying data, are:

Ineffective Thermoregulation—RESOLVED. Mr. Wilson's temperature is stable and is not fluctuating between Hypothermia and Hyperthermia.

Constipation—RESOLVED. Mr. Wilson has had two bowel movements. His fluid intake has increased and he is on a soft diet

Dysfunctional Ventilatory Weaning Response—RESOLVED. Mr. Wilson is off of the ventilator and his respirations are regular and unlabored.

Unilateral Neglect—CONTINUE. Mr. Wilson still ignores his affected side and does not attend to safety or self care on that side. Additionally he leaves food on the plate on the affected side,. The target date needs to be changed and the nursing actions continued.

Spiritual Distress—REVISED. Mrs. Wilson has expressed relief and peace about the situation and is seeking support from the church.

Change to Family Coping, Potential for Growth (Page 730). Have students identify new expected outcomes, target date, and nursing actions.

FOLLOW-UP

MR. JOSEPH WILSON

Mr. Wilson has now been in the hospital for eight days. His temperature has remained stable for the last three days ranging from 98 degree F to 99.2 degrees F. His pulse is 84 and regular and his blood pressure is 130/86. After two attempts to wean Mr. Wilson from the ventilator, the third attempt was successful. Mr. Wilson's endotracheal tube was removed yesterday and his respirations are 18 and regular.

Mr. Wilson's feeding tube was also removed yesterday. He was started on a clear liquid progressive diet. He tolerated the liquids well. His intake was 2500 ml yesterday including the I.V. fluids. He ate a soft diet this morning. but left the food on the right side of the plate. His I.V. is scheduled to be discontinued today. Mr. Wilson had a fairly hard, well-formed stool two days ago and a soft, well- formed stool early this morning. He continues on Dulcolax tab 1 at bedtime.

Mr. Wilson can talk now that the endotracheal tube has been removed. However, his mouth pulls to the left and he is occasionally unsure of the words. He is oriented to time, place, and person. Thought processes and both short-term and long-term memory are intact. Deep tendon reflexes on the right side are diminished and he responds to sharp pain by facial grimace and attempts to withdraw arm or leg from the source. Muscle tone is returning. Mr. Wilson continues to ignore his right side and needs assistance in positioning his right arm and leg and in caring for his right side.

Mr. and Mrs. Wilson have had several opportunities to talk since the endotracheal tube has been removed. Mr. Wilson expresses happiness to be alive and promises to wear his seat belt from now on. He does not blame the drunk driver and believes that God must have a reason for involving him in this accident. Mr. Wilson requested that his minister come and talk with both of them and they have prayed together. Mrs. Wilson's mood reflects relief and she no longer blames God for the accident. Mrs. Wilson has gone back to church and is receiving support from the women's group of the church.

Mr. and Mrs. Wilson have talked with the physician about the long-term treatment plan and are anxious to begin the rehabilitation process. The occupational therapist and physical therapist have been consulted and Mr. Wilson is scheduled for treatments today. Mrs. Wilson will attend these sessions so that she can participate in Mr. Wilson's care. Mr. Wilson has expressed interest in learning new job-related skills.

MR. DAVID PATTERSON

David Patterson is an 18-year-old man who requested an appointment at the Nursing Center because "I just can't seem to keep my grades up and my girlfriend is worried about me." The initial session with David provided the following information.

David describes himself as an average student who has to work hard to maintain "average" grades. He has maintained a GPA of 3.9 as a chemistry/premed major in his first year at the University. In the last four months he reports his grades have been mostly B's and he is very concerned about this. He comes from an upper middle class family where he is the youngest of four children. David's family lives 500 miles away and this is the longest he has lived away from his family. He visited with his family at the semester break and plans a week at home before he starts summer school. His parents and siblings all have established themselves in their careers. He feels as if he is failing his family by not maintaining a 4.0 GPA. He reports having tried everything to get his grades up and "it just isn't working. I no longer have control, it is in the hands of my professors." He indicated he was ready to drop out of school and take a blue collar job when his girlfriend convinced him to come talk with someone first.

David reports that his girlfriend's concern evolved from an incident that happened the previous weekend. They had been at a party at his fraternity house and had been drinking. He has no memory for what happened except that his girlfriend told him he began throwing the furniture when she indicated that he had had enough to drink and she left because she was afraid he might hurt her. David indicates that he has been drinking socially since junior high school. His father would drink every night from the time he got home from work until bedtime and David does not want to be like his dad but is afraid not to drink because he thinks the guys in his fraternity will reject him if he does not party with them. When he starts drinking he just cannot stop. David is very remorseful about what happened the other night and starts crying while saying, "I just don't know what to do, I have no control over it once I get started." He has not talked with anyone about these concerns because he is afraid they will laugh and reject him for being an "egghead."

At the end of the session David indicates an interest in getting help but is not sure that he has a drinking problem. He is also very concerned about losing the support of his fraternity brothers if he acts differently.

NURSING DIAGNOSES ACCORDING TO PATTERNS

HEALTH PERCEPTION-HEALTH MANAGEMENT PATTERN

Health Seeking Behaviors (Page 37)

Defining Characteristics Present

Indicates desire for help by coming for appointment and indicating an interest in getting help at the end of the session.

Indicates several times that he just did not know what to do to change his situation

Indicated concern that social environment supports his drinking even though he recognizes that this is not what he wants to do

Girlfriend informed him of resource (Nursing Center) and he is new to this community

NOTE: STUDENTS MAY WISH TO USE DIAGNOSIS OF ALTERED HEALTH MAINTENANCE (Page 29); HOWEVER, THE MAJOR DEFINING CHARACTERISTICS FIT BEST WITH HEALTH SEEKING BEHAVIORS.

NUTRITIONAL-METABOLIC PATTERN

No diagnoses related to this pattern. The students may want to use Altered Nutrition based on previous experience with clients experiencing problems with chemical abuse but, the data does not support this diagnosis at this time. This would be an area for future assessment.

ELIMINATION PATTERN

No diagnoses related to this pattern

ACTIVITY-EXERCISE PATTERN

No diagnoses related to this pattern

SLEEP-REST PATTERN

No diagnoses related to this pattern

COGNITIVE-PERCEPTUAL PATTERN

Decisional Conflict (page 426)

Defining Characteristics Present

Wants to change his drinking patterns but is concerned about maintaining relationships
with peers

Not ready to commit to one choice or alteration in lifestyle at the end of the first session

Remorseful about drinking behavior. Tearful while talking about this behavior

Does not want to be like his Dad but afraid of the reaction of his peers if he does stop
drinking

Not sure he really has a problem, thinks he may be thought to be over reacting by his
friends (may be called an "egghead")

NOTE: STUDENTS MAY WISH TO USE DIAGNOSIS OF KNOWLEDGE DEFICIT
AND/ OR ALTERED THOUGHT PROCESS (PAGES 439 AND 476) ; HOWEVER,
THE MAJOR DEFINING CHARACTERISTICS FIT BEST WITH DECISIONAL
CONFLICT.

SELF-PERCEPTION AND SELF-CONCEPT PATTERN

Powerlessness (page 545)

Defining Characteristics Present

Verbal expressions of having no control or influence over situation

Verbal expressions of having no control or influence over outcome

Apathy

Self Esteem Disturbance (page 553)

Defining Characteristics Present

Self negating verbalization

Expressions of shame/guilt

Evaluates self as unable to deal with events

Rationalizes away/rejects positive feedback and exaggerates negative feedback about self

Hesitant to try new things/situation

Hypersensitive to slight or criticism

Rationalizing personal failures

NOTE: STUDENTS MAY WISH TO USE THE DIAGNOSIS OF HOPELESSNESS

(PAGE 524); THE DATA MORE ACCURATELY FIT THE DEFINING

CHARACTERISTICS FOR POWERLESSNESS.

ROLE-RELATIONSHIP PATTERN

Violence, Risk for (page 661)

Risk Factors Present

Destroyed property when approached by girlfriend about drinking

Alcohol abuse; history of at least one blackout while drinking

Feels his professors are in control of his academic achievement

Expressed increased discomfort (anxiety) with his school performance and his inability to change the situation

Feels he cannot share his feelings with those he perceives to be his support system

Many self-deprecatory statements

Girlfriend indicated she was afraid of him while he was drinking

NOTE: STUDENTS MAY WISH TO USE DIAGNOSIS OF ALTERED ROLE PERFORMANCE (PAGE 631) DUE TO THE CONCERNS THAT ARE VERBALIZED BY THE CLIENT ABOUT HIS PERCEIVED ABILITIES TO PERFORM HIS ROLE AS STUDENT; HOWEVER, THE DEFINING CHARACTERISTICS FOR THIS DIAGNOSIS ARE NOT COMPLETELY SUPPORTED AT THE 70% LEVEL BY THE DATA. THE DIAGNOSIS OF SELF-ESTEEM DISTURBANCE PROVIDES A MORE COMPREHENSIVE USE OF THE DATA AND THE DEFINING CHARACTERISTICS ARE MET.

SEXUALITY-REPRODUCTIVE PATTERN

No diagnoses related to this pattern

COPING-STRESS TOLERANCE PATTERN

No diagnoses related to this pattern; however, students may want to use Ineffective Individual Coping or Defensive Individual Coping (page 735) based on the client's desire to give up. This response is based more on his perception that his actions cannot influence the situation; therefore, the diagnosis of Powerlessness is more accurate.

VALUE-BELIEF PATTERN

176

No diagnoses related to this pattern

EXPECTED OUTCOMES AND TARGET DATES

Have students write own expected outcomes first then compare and contrast to the expected outcomes in the book. Health Seeking Behavior, page 37; Decisional Conflict, page 426 ; Powerlessness, page 545 ; Risk for Violence, page 661; and Self-Esteem Disturbance, page 553 .

NURSING ACTIONS

Refer students to appropriate pages in book. Have them select nursing actions pertinent for David and individualize these orders for David's age and condition.

EVALUATION

Use the follow-up on the next page. Again, have students group data according to each diagnosis. Refer the students to the appropriate evaluation decision flow sheet in the book. Have the students list the data collected as it related to each expected outcome and them make decisions as to whether they are going to record REVISE, CONTINUE, or RESOLVED for each diagnosis.

The most appropriate decisions based on the data are:

Health Seeking Behavior—RESOLVED. David is now involved with health care systems that will assist him in moving toward higher levels of health. Students may want to use CONTINUE here because of David's response to his use of alcohol; however, the data does not meet the defining criteria for this diagnosis. The data related to the alcoholism supports a new diagnosis that will be later presented.

Decisional Conflict—RESOLVED. David has made choices related to his relationships with his peers and is maintaining a healthy life-style with his new assertive skills. Again students may want to CONTINUE this diagnosis due to the data about the use of alcohol; however, the data does not support the defining characteristics.

Powerlessness—RESOLVED. Davis is taking assertive action in his own behalf and verbalizes a new sense of control over his life.

Self-Esteem Disturbance—CONTINUE. David continues to demonstrate self-deprecatory thinking and has difficulty accepting positive feedback. He also expresses a great deal of guilt and does not feel confident in new situations so he continues to have difficulty in new situations.

Violence, Risk for—RESOLVED. David has not had any angry outbursts since he has quit drinking. This diagnosis may be addressed again if David resumes his previous drinking patterns.

As stated earlier Decisional Conflict and Health Seeking Behaviors have been RESOLVED or the students may choose to use REVISED and **add** the diagnosis of Ineffective Individual Coping: Defensive . This diagnosis is supported by David's inability to acknowledge that he has difficulty with alcohol regardless of the fact that he still has the desire to drink and he places the responsibility for his drinking behavior on others in his environment. He is also having difficulty reality-testing which he demonstrates by comparing his drinking patterns to his father's and by denying the degree of difficulty alcohol caused in his life. David is also demonstrating difficulty in following up on treatment.

MR. DAVID PATTERSON

David has been coming to the Nursing Center once a week for one hour sessions for two months. During this time he has enrolled in an assertiveness training class at the campus counseling center. He indicates that he is more comfortable telling his friends at the fraternity house that he does not want to drink with them and has not had a drink for six weeks in spite of his concern that they will reject him.

He has acknowledged that his behavior can have an impact on his future and is practicing relaxation exercises as a way to cope with the stress of school. David acknowledges that he still feels as though he has failed his family and cannot accept the fact that he has made progress in the past two months because he still makes Bs at times. He has not had a violent outburst since he has quit drinking. He does admit that he still wants to drink especially when he feels a great deal of pressure from school or when his friends want him to party with them. He can control this urge by spending time with his girlfriend or by calling her.

He states very strongly that he does not have a problem with alcohol and that when he did get into trouble with his drinking it was because his friends forced him to drink or because of the pressure he was feeling at school. When this issue comes up during therapy sessions his speech becomes more rapid and he indicates that his Dad drinks more than he does and his Dad is successful so there is no problem with alcohol. Several times he has agreed to attend a campus group of Alcoholics Anonymous but has not followed through saying that he has done it on his own for two months and he does not need help in this area. David expresses an interest in continuing counseling at the Nursing Center to work on his coping behaviors.

CASE STUDY 9

MR. ROGER DALTON

Roger Dalton is a 35-year-old white mane recently discharged from the hospital after being treated for Pneumocystitis carinii pneumonia. He is HIV positive and has experienced several hospitalizations in the past year. He is now being managed at home. John, a 36-year-old man, is his long-time companion. John is the primary care giver for Roger. On your first home visit, you gather the following information.

S: Roger complains of feeling hot and cold, short of breath, tired, and weak. John reports that Roger is having trouble sleeping and sometimes doesn't recognize him. John is particularly worried that he cannot get Roger to eat. John also reports that Roger's condition has deteriorated since the recent bout with pneumocystis. "He can't do anything for himself anymore...he just wets the bed."

O: House is cluttered by equipment and supplies to care for Roger. Urine-and feces-soiled linen and clothes are in a pile on floor in bathroom. Smell of urine and feces in bedroom and bathroom. Roger is thin, weak, and withdrawn. John is anxious and attentive to Roger's needs.

Lab drawn during hospitalization indicates a low CD_4 lymphocyte count and thrombocytopenia.

Vitals: T-101 degrees F orally, BP-110/60, P-100, R-20

Skin: Diaphoretic, generalized xerosis, multiple small bruises on forearms and legs

Neck: Generalized cervical lymphadenopathy

Mouth: Gums swollen, plaque on teeth

Chest: Cough productive of yellow sputum, crackles present at lung bases bilaterally

GI: Incontinent of diarrheal stool 3-4 times per day

Neurological: Difficult for Roger to follow directions, he is very slow to respond to questions or commands, cranial nerves 2-12 grossly intact. Unable to perform cerebellar tests, weakness in all extremities, unable to walk without support due to ataxia and weakness. Does not know date and time, does not recognize John.

During the exam, John talks to you about his difficulty in keeping the house, caring for all of Roger's needs, and the "enormous" debts Roger's illness has caused. John wonders if there is any source of assistance to manage John at home. During the exam, Roger repeatedly strikes at you and John yelling, "Leave me alone." John becomes visibly upset and leaves the room. After calming Roger, you talk to John privately. John tells you:

"I don't know what to do. I can't take care of Roger.I don't have enough money, time, or energy. I will have to quit my job. I can't take it when Roger doesn't recognize me. We used to be so close. I can't go out anymore. Many of our friends are afraid to be seen with us now, They won't even call. His family calls to see how he is, but they don't offer any help. He won't eat, his skin is so fragile, it bruises and he gets sores that won't heal. I am so worried and upset. I just don't know what to do."

NURSING DIAGNOSES ACCORDING TO PATTERNS

HEALTH PERCEPTION-HEALTH MANAGEMENT PATTERN

Protection, Altered (Page 85)

Defining Characteristics Present

Deficient immunity—HIV positive, low CD4 lymphocytes, pneumocystitis carinii

Impaired healing—"he gets sores that won't heal"

Altered clotting—thrombocytopenia, bruises on forearms and lower extremities

Neurosensory alterations—incontinent, unable to perform cerebellar functions, ataxia, does not recognize care giver

Chilling, Perspiring, Dyspnea, Cough, Restlessness, Insomnia, Fatigue,

Anorexia, Weakness, Disorientation

NOTE: RISK FOR INFECTION IS OFTEN A COMPANION DIAGNOSIS (Page 43)

NUTRITIONAL-METABOLIC PATTERN

No diagnoses in this pattern

ELIMINATION PATTERN

No diagnoses in this pattern

ACTIVITY-EXERCISE PATTERN

Home Maintenance Management, Impaired (page 344)

Defining Characteristics Present

Subjective: Household members express difficulty in maintaining their home in a comfortable fashion—John's statements

Household requests assistance with home maintenance—John's questions regarding the availability of assistance

Household members describe outstanding debts or financial crisis—John describes "enormous debts", "I don't have enough money." "I will have to quit my job."

Objective: Disorderly surroundings—house is cluttered by equipment and supplies

Unwashed or unavailable cooking equipment, clothes, or linen—urine- and feces- soiled clothing and linen in bathroom

Accumulation of dirt, food wastes, or hygienic wastes—urine- and feces-soiled clothing and linen in bathroom

Overtaxed family members, e.g., exhausted, anxious—John is anxious; "I don't know what to do. I can't take care of Roger."

Self Care Deficit: Toileting (Page 371)

Defining Characteristics Present

Unable to get to toilet or commode—weakness, ataxia, disorientation; diarrheal stools

Unable to manipulate clothing for toileting—weakness, ataxia, disorientation; "He cannot do anything for himself anymore."

Unable to carry out proper toilet hygiene—soiled clothing and linen in bathroom

SLEEP-REST PATTERN

No diagnoses in this pattern

COGNITIVE-PERCEPTUAL PATTERN

No diagnoses in this pattern

SELF- PERCEPTION AND SELF-CONCEPT PATTERN

No diagnoses in this pattern

ROLE-RELATIONSHIP PATTERN

<u>Caregiver Role Strain</u> (Page 573)

Defining Characteristics Present

Do not have enough resources to provide the care needed—John states, "I don't have enough money, time, or energy."

Find it hard to do specific caregiving activities—unable to keep up with incontinence, oral hygiene, and so forth.

Worry about such things as the care receiver's health and emotional state—"He won't eat, his skin is so fragile."

Feel that caregiving interferes with other important roles in their lives—John states, "I can't go out anymore." "I will have to quit my job."

Feel loss because the care receiver is like a different person compared to before caregiving began—John states, "I can't take it when Roger doesn't recognize me. We used to be so close."

Feel family conflict around issues of providing care—"His family calls to see how he is, but they don't offer any help."

NOTE: STUDENTS MAY WISH TO USE THE DIAGNOSIS OF INEFFECTIVE
INDIVIDUAL COPING. THE DIFFERENTIATING FACTOR IS WHETHER OR
NOT THE INDIVIDUAL IS INVOLVED IN A CAREGIVING ROLE OR NOT.

Social Isolation (page 645)

Defining Characteristics Present

Absence of supportive significant other(s)--John is supportive, but overwhelmed; family is
distant; friends are afraid, projects hostility in voice, behavior—repeatedly strikes at
examiner and caregiver; yelling, "Leave me at alone."

Seeks to be alone—yells, "Leave me alone."

Evidence of physical/mental handicap or altered state of wellness—HIV positive with
decreased lymphocytes and opportunistic infection; disoriented; decreased cerebellar
functions; incontinence

NOTE: IN ADDITION TO THE FIVE DIAGNOSES GIVEN, STUDENT MAY ALSO
SELECT DIARRHEA, INCONTINENCE, OR HYPERTHERMIA. WHILE ALL OF
THESE ARE PRESENT IN THE CASE, IT IS IMPORTANT TO RECOGNIZE THAT
THEY ARE ALSO INDICATIONS OF BROADER DIAGNOSES.

EXPECTED OUTCOMES AND TARGET DATES

Have students write own expected outcomes first and then compare and contrast to
the expected outcomes in the book. Altered Protection page 85; Caregiver Role Strain
page 573; Impaired Home Maintenance Management page 344; Self-Care Deficit page
371; and Social Isolation page 645.

NURSING ACTIONS

Refer students to appropriate pages in book. Have them select nursing actions appropriate for Roger and John and individualize these actions according to Roger's and John's particular situation.

EVALUATION

Use follow-up on next page. Again, have students group data according to each diagnosis. Refer the student to the appropriate evaluation decision flow sheet in the book. Have the students list the data collected as it related to each expected outcome and then make decisions as to whether they are going to record REVISE, CONTINUE, or RESOLVED for each diagnosis.

The most appropriate decisions, based upon the accompanying data are:

Altered Protection—CONTINUE. Although improvement in diarrhea and cough, Roger's immune system remains compromised.

Caregiver Role Strain—RESOLVED. Roger and John are now receiving more financial and physical support.

Impaired Home Maintenance Management—RESOLVED. Roger and John have found ways to meet these needs.

Social Isolation—CONTINUE. Although Rogers' family and friends are becoming more involved; this diagnosis is still appropriate.

Self-Care Deficit—CONTINUE. John still needs to assist Roger in toileting functions.

FOLLOW-UP

MR. ROGER DALTON

Since the last visit to Roger and John, they have received the assistance of a home health aid who visits daily. Roger's sister and John's brother have also helped out a few days a month so that John can continue working. John reports he is now able to care for Roger adequately with this help. Both Roger and John are much more relaxed. Roger has received treatment from his physician for his cough and diarrhea. Episodes of incontinence are decreasing, although Roger still requires assistance with toileting. John reports that Roger recognizes him "most of the time" now. John attends a support group weekly. Roger attends when he is feeling well. He has attended all but two sessions with John. Both report that they are making new friends. Roger has been approved for financial assistance. Part of John's salary can now be dedicated to debt reduction.

You note that the house is much more efficiently organized; the smell of urine and feces is absent. There is no dirty linen or laundry present. Roger is alert and oriented and responds to questions. John reports that Roger often sleeps through the night and he is now eating six small meals daily. Roger remains ataxic.

CASE STUDY 10

MR. CHARLES DEAN

Mr. Charles Dean is a 78-year-old retired farmer, admitted to the Special Care Unit of Golden Ages Nursing Home with the medical diagnosis of Senile Dementia Alzheimer's Type (SDAT). During the admission interview Mr. Dean's wife Rose tells the nurse she can no longer care for Charles at home. "It's like he's a stranger. He usually thinks I'm his mother and not his wife." Mrs. Dean reports financial problems due to a large number of checks drawn on their account with the money missing. "Charles handled all our bills and expenses, I don't know where the money went." Mrs. Dean describes the main problems she has encountered with caring for Charles as problems with toileting, verbal and physical aggression, and wandering. She states she has to have Charles wear adult diapers. "He doesn't use the bathroom when he needs to." She also states that Charles is increasingly restless and sleeps only for brief periods. "He's up at all hours walking around the house and I can't get him to stay awake during the day." Recently Charles has become physically aggressive, especially when there are visitors in the house, and when the TV is playing. His primary physician has prescribed Haldol 0.5 mg P.O. B.I.D.

Mr. Dean's admission vital signs are T. 97 degrees orally, P. 80 and regular, R. 16, B.P. 138/84. He is hard of hearing and uses glasses for reading. He is 5' 10" tall and weighs 135 pounds. He is pale, thin, has sluggish skin turgor, dark circles under his eyes, and is easily distracted. The nurse also notes numerous bruises on his extremities, in various stages of healing, along with decreased muscle tone especially in the upper extremities. The abdominal exam reveals hyperactive bowel sounds and Mr. Dean grimaces when his abdomen is lightly palpated. During the mental status exam he is unable to remember 3 items after 3 minutes have passed. He cannot interpret the proverb, "a stitch in time saves nine," and cannot state what city or state he lives in. Admission blood work reveals a decreased Hct., Hgb., iron-binding capacity, and serum Albumin. During the first week post admission, the nursing staff notes numerous problems related to Mr. Dean's care. At mealtimes, Mr. Dean will begin eating and abruptly leave the table. He states that the meals "taste like slop." He will wander on the unit and into other resident's rooms. He frequently states he is looking for the car keys and has to go home. He accuses other residents of stealing his things. "I came here with all of my northings and you've got them." While prompted to toilet every 3-4 hours, Mr. Dean still has episodes of incontinence. On night rounds, the nursing staff has found Mr. Dean using the waste paper basket as a urinal. The night staff also reports that Mr. Dean wanders at all hours, attempts to leave the unit and tries to get into bed with his roommate. When asked to return to his own bed, Mr. Dean often ignores the staff or threatens to "have the mannerings get you." The nursing staff on the morning shift has noticed Mr. Dean is very tired in the morning. He complains of "too many children in the house at nighttime" and insists that staff stay out of his room, so he can keep his business going.

NURSING DIAGNOSES ACCORDING TO PATTERNS

HEALTH PERCEPTION-HEALTH MANAGEMENT PATTERN

Risk for Trauma (Page 50)

Defining Characteristics Present (Internal)

History of previous trauma—multiple bruises in various stages of healing

Cognitive Difficulties—patient's behavior and wife's statement

Lack of Safety Precautions—wandering, aggressiveness

Decreased hearing—nurse's exam

Fatigue—wife's statement; sleep pattern

NUTRITIONAL-METABOLIC PATTERN

Altered Nutrition: Less than Body Requirements (Page 163)

Defining Characteristics Present

Body weight greater than 20% under ideal—weighs 138 pounds

Inadequate food intake (less than RDA)--wife's statement, nurses' observation

Anemia—Hct and Hgb measurements

Decreased serum Albumin—lab results

Decreased Iron binding capacity—lab results

Aversion to eating—wife's comments, patient's comments

Self reported altered taste sensation—"tastes like slop"

Hyperactive bowel sounds—nurse's exam

Lack of interest in food—wife's statements

Pale conjunctiva—nurse's exam

Poor muscle tone—nurse's exam

Abdominal pain—grimacing at light abdominal palpation

ELIMINATION PATTERN

<u>Altered</u> <u>Urinary</u> <u>Elimination</u> <u>Pattern</u>: <u>Functional</u> <u>Incontinence</u> (Page 229)

Defining Characteristics Present

Loss of urine before reaching appropriate receptacle—wife's statement

Unpredictable voiding pattern—nurse's observation

ACTIVITY-EXERCISE PATTERN

No diagnoses related to this pattern

SLEEP-REST PATTERN

<u>Sleep</u> <u>Pattern</u> <u>Disturbance</u> (Page 397)

Defining Characteristics Present

Dark circles under eyes—nurse's observation

Irritable—wife's and nurse's observation

Interrupted sleep—wife's and patient's statements, nurse's observation

Early morning awakening—nurse's observation

Napping during day—wife's comments

COGNITIVE-PERCEPTUAL PATTERN

Altered Thought Process (Page 476)

Defining Characteristics Present

Easily distracted, Inaccurate interpretation of environment—patient's statements, nurse's
observation

Memory deficits, poor short term memory—wife's statements, nurse's mental status exam

Hypervigiliance in regard to room and possessions—patient's statements

SELF-PERCEPTION AND SELF-CONCEPT PATTERN

No diagnoses in this pattern

ROLE-RELATIONSHIP PATTERN

No diagnoses in this pattern

SEXUALITY-REPRODUCTIVE PATTERN

No diagnoses in this pattern

COPING-STRESS TOLERANCE PATTERN

No diagnoses in this pattern

VALUE-BELIEF PATTERN

No diagnoses in this pattern

EXPECTED OUTCOMES AND TARGET DATES

Have students write own expected outcomes first and then compare and contrast to
the expected outcomes in the book. Risk for Trauma, page 50 ; Altered Nutrition: Less
than Body Requirements, page 163 ; Altered Urinary Elimination Pattern: Functional

Incontinence, page 229; Sleep Pattern Disturbance, page 397 ; and Altered Thought Process, page 476 .

NURSING ACTIONS

Refer students to appropriate pages in book. Have them select nursing actions appropriate for Mr. Dean and individualize these actions according to Mr. Dean's particular diagnoses and developmental level.

EVALUATION

Use follow-up on next page. Again, have students group data according to each diagnosis. Refer the student to the appropriate evaluation decision flow sheet in the book. Have the students list the data collected as it related to each expected outcome and then make decisions as to whether they are going to record REVISE, CONTINUE, or RESOLVED for each diagnosis.

The most appropriate decisions based on the accompanying data are:

Risk for Trauma—CONTINUE and change target date. Mr. Dean still has the defining characteristics for this diagnosis.

Altered Nutrition: Less than Body Requirements—REVISE to Risk for. Mr. Dean is gaining weight and consuming meals with staff prompting.

Altered Urinary Elimination Pattern: Functional Incontinence—CONTINUE and change target date. Mr. Dean has fewer incontinent episodes but the problem remains.

Sleep Pattern Disturbance—RESOLVED. Mr. Dean no longer has the defining characteristics for this diagnosis.

FOLLOW-UP

MR. CHARLES DEAN

Mr. Dean has remained on the Special Care Unit for two months. He continues to be easily distracted. There are no longer dark circles under his eyes and he rarely naps during the daytime. His wife reports he now enjoys eating goodies from home and having the grandchildren come to visit. Nutritionally, he is now, with prompting from the staff, eating small, frequent meals and consumes between meal nutritional supplements. He has gained 10 pounds in the past 2 months.

He currently participates in a number of group activities including morning exercises and chapel services as well as Reminiscing Time. The night staff reports that Mr. Dean is usually in bed most of the night and falls asleep soon after awakening for toileting. As a result of every 3-hour toileting, Mr. Dean no longer requires adult diapers. The staff have noted several instances of nocturnal incontinence when Mr. Dean takes fluids after 8:30 p.m. While there are fewer episodes of aggression noted, he is still concerned when staff attempt to enter his room and his mental status exams have shown no improvement.

Altered Thought Process—CONTINUE and change target date. Mr. Dean still has the defining characteristics for this diagnosis.

PART VI --TRANSPARENCY MASTERS

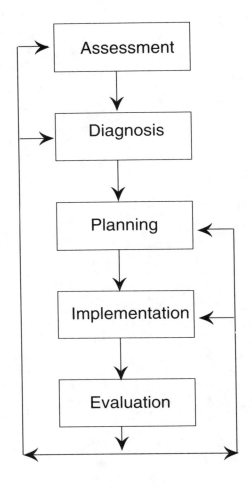

Fig. 1-1 Nursing Process Flowchart

PATTERN	DESCRIPTION
Health Perception- Health Management	The patient's awareness of personal health and well-being; health practices; understanding of how health practices contribute to health status.
Nutritional-Metabolic	The patient's description of food and fluid intake; relationship of intake to metabolic needs; include indicators of ineffectual nutrition on metabolic functioning, e.g., healing.
Elimination	Description of all routes and routines of output. Includes any aids to excretion.
Activity-Exercise	Patient's overall activities of daily living, including recreational activity.
Sleep-Rest	Patient's 24-hour routine of rest, relaxation, and sleep.
Cognitive-Perceptual	Cognitive functional performance and sensory performance.
Self-Perception Self-Concept	Patient's self-assessment; attitudes, ability, worth; verbal and nonverbal communication.
Role-Relationship	Patient's assessment of all roles, related responsibilities, and interrelatedness between these factors and other people.
Sexuality-Reproductive	Satisfaction-dissatisfaction with sexuality. Any dysfunction in sexuality or reproduction.
Coping-Stress Tolerance	Effectiveness or noneffectiveness in dealing with difficult situations; how handles; reaction to; support available.
Value-Belief	Ideas held in esteem by patient. guiding principles for overall life-style.

Table 1-3   Functional Health Patterns (From Gordon[22], p. 2, with permission).

PATTERN	DESCRIPTION
EXCHANGING	To give, relinquish, or lose something while receiving something in return; the substitution of one element for another; the reciprocal act of giving and receiving.
COMMUNICATING	To converse; to impart, confer, or transmit thoughts, feelings, or information, internally or externally, verbally or nonverbally.
RELATING	To connect, to establish a link between, to stand in some association to another thing, person, or place; to be borne or thrust in between things.
VALUING	To be concerned about, to care; the worth or worthiness; the relative status of a thing, or the estimate in which it is held, according to its real or supposed worth, usefulness, or importance; one's opinion of like for a person or thing; to equate in importance.
CHOOSING	To select between alternatives; the action of selecting or exercising preference in regard to a matter in which one is a free agent; to determine in favor of a course; to decide in accordance with inclinations.
MOVING	To change the place or position of a body or any member of the body; to put and/or keep in motion; to provoke an excretion or discharge; the urge to action or to do something; leave in; to take action.
PERCEIVING	To apprehend with the mind; to become aware of by the senses; to apprehend what is not open or present to observation; to take in fully or adequately.
KNOWING	To recognize or acknowledge a thing or person; to be familiar with by experience or through information or report; to be cognizant of something through observation, inquiry, or information; to be conversant with a body of facts, principles, or methods of action; to understand.
FEELING	To experience a consciousness, sensation, apprehension, or sense; to be consciously or emotionally affected by a fact, event, or state.

Table 1-4   Human Response Patterns (From Fitzpatrick, JJ: Taxonomy II: Definitions and development. In Carroll-Johnson, RM (ed): Classification of Nursing Diagnosis: Proceedings of the Ninth Conference. Lippincott, Philadelphia, 1991).

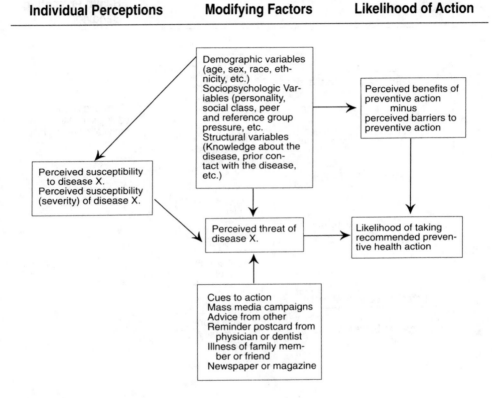

Figure. 2-1 The Health Belief Model. (From Becker, MH, et al: Selected psychosocial models and correlates of individual health-related behaviors. Medical Care 15:27, 1977 [Supplement], with permission.)

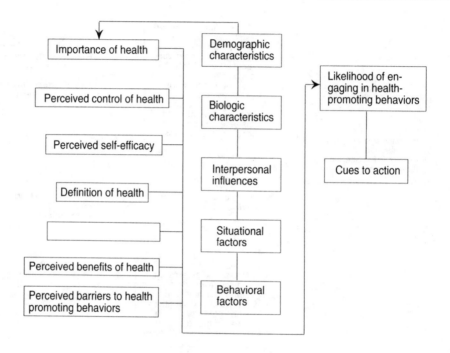

Figure. 2-2 Health Promotion Model. (From Pender,[6] p58, with permission.)

INSTRUCTIONS FOR NEXT TRANSPARENCY MASTERS

The next 3 transparencies have to be used in exact sequence according to the number in the upper right hand corner. These transparencies, when used in the proper order, assist you to teach the student how to follow the evaluation flow charts in the textbook as well as teaching them how to construct their own evaluation flow charts. By placing transparency 2 on top of 1, then 3 on top of these two, you can focus on selected parts of the flow chart without overwhelming the student with too much information.

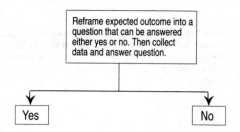

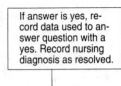

If answer is yes, re-
cord data used to an-
swer question with a
yes. Record nursing
diagnosis as resolved.

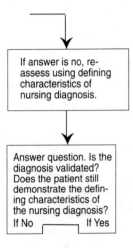

If answer is no, re-
assess using defining
characteristics of
nursing diagnosis.

Answer question. Is the
diagnosis validated?
Does the patient still
demonstrate the defin-
ing characteristics of
the nursing diagnosis?
If No   If Yes

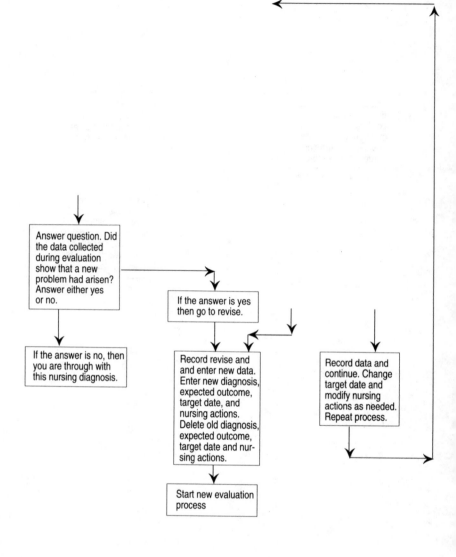

Answer question. Did the data collected during evaluation show that a new problem had arisen? Answer either yes or no.

If the answer is yes then go to revise.

If the answer is no, then you are through with this nursing diagnosis.

Record revise and and enter new data. Enter new diagnosis, expected outcome, target date, and nursing actions. Delete old diagnosis, expected outcome, target date and nursing actions.

Record data and continue. Change target date and modify nursing actions as needed. Repeat process.

Start new evaluation process